Skin Care

The Truth About Caring for Darker Skin

(The Ultimate Diy Guide on How to Make Organic Toners)

Donald Godoy

Published By **Elena Holly**

Donald Godoy

All Rights Reserved

Skin Care: The Truth About Caring for Darker Skin (The Ultimate Diy Guide on How to Make Organic Toners)

ISBN   978-1-77485-687-1

Legal & Disclaimer

Table Of Contents

Introduction

Many people believe that making your own cosmetics from scratch is a lengthy and difficult procedure. Today there is convenience everywhere and are able to discover a variety of commercially-produced products. But the issue is that very few consumers doubt the ingredients in the cosmetics themselves. It's becoming increasingly difficult to find organic cosmetics because everything we buy is mass-produced and designed to last a long shelf time. This means that there are usually harmful, unneeded ingredients in store-bought cosmetics product that could lead to issues in the short or long term. Making your own health products does not just eliminate concerns about the ingredients you're putting on your skin, but also provides an individual, unique touch on your own creations.

Organic, Natural, and Pure are terms that are used by many companies in order to promote their goods. They don't say that a variety of preservatives or chemical compounds of similar nature are also incorporated into their "natural" mixtures. A lot of people are aware that even though the products claim to be organic according to the labels, there's more in these items than meets the eye.

This book you'll learn how to make natural beauty products using all natural components.

Before we start our journey, we must be aware of the best practices and rules. Cleaning is essential when using homemade skincare products. Make sure you clean your workspace, all tools and equipment involved and the containers that are used to store your cosmetics. Since the reason for making natural skin care products at home are to provide nourishment to your skin in a natural way, it's vital that there's no bacteria or mold growing within our products.

Within this book, you'll discover a assortment of recipes. Before choosing one recipe that you would like to create for yourself, you need to determine what kind that skin is yours.

There are generally five types of skin that comprise regular skin, oily, dry and combination skin, and sensitive skin. Normal skin is even toned and is generally soft. Skin that is oily tends to be oily and shiny on the forehead and around the nose region. Dry skin is often rough, leaving rough skin. Combination skin can be oily in certain parts (around the nose, forehead and the chin) while dry in others. The sensitive skin can suffer from burning or itchy sensations.

The reactions are typically due to other skincare products, therefore it is recommended to be aware of what products could be responsible for the reaction and then stay clear of these products again in the near future.

Once you've determined the type of skin you have There are a variety of recipes in this book that fall into every category. I suggest you explore a few of the recipes and decide which one is best for you!

Chapter 1: Making Soap Making

Many people have likely never imagined they could create soap. It looks to take an entire day and would be a hassle however in reality it's surprisingly fast and simple. Even your grandmother could manage it. This is why you should think about creating soap in your home to conquer any fears you may have about the process.

After you've finished studying this book The urge to create soap at home be overwhelming. It's a good idea, but I encourage you to accept the feeling. Making soap isn't just an enjoyable activity however, it also offers positive health and economic benefits. There are social, health and economic aspects that demonstrate the importance of soap production.

Benefits of soap Making

Here are a few of the major benefits making soap at home:

It is your final decision maker about what ingredients to use.

The great thing about making soap is that you're in total control. You get to choose the recipe you'd prefer to make as well as select the ingredients you prefer. You can rock your boat however you'd like and in the manner that you like. From the design of the soap, to the color , and even the inclination to a certain type of scent, you're free to alter your homemade soap to suit your preferences. In addition, you can decide about the texture, amount of soap it creates and much more.

Additionally, when making the soaps, you'll have something exciting to get excited about. There is nothing like that sensation of tingling which makes you feel happy, particularly when you can inform your pals "I did this."

I am sure that with a thinking and a bit of imagination and some initiative soaps can be wonderful.

* You can turn it into a profitable business

Many soapmakers have launched and expanded their businesses out of something that may have started as a pastime. With limited resources and a vision to follow the right goals, soap makers have managed to turn more customers to customers and achieve an impressive return on their investment, to the point that they're employed and earn enough revenue to support themselves and their staff.

Soap manufacturing is a fantastic opportunity for investors who are interested in investing. There is no market issue. Most people use soap on a daily to daily basis. It is possible to sell soaps to anyone who has even the slightest desire for the product you've made. It may be your family members or at local markets and restaurants, hospitals and school fairs, or even via the internet. The market waiting to take advantage of your product is huge and, with the correct method of operation, your business will grow.

As time passes your knowledge increases and with that type of advancement, you're capable of converting your small investment into a massive business that will eventually make you a good revenue. You can also go further by educating your peers and expanding your business.

It's a good alternative

Based on the most recent survey the latest study suggests that glycerin, petrochemicals and a variety of other alkaline substances that are available in nearly all stores that sell soaps can be responsible for skin irritations. Petrochemicals are absorbed into the skin through the absorption process. They then pile into the tissues beneath. As time passes the body can suffer from complications, such as severe brain and liver damage. Additionally, high-alkaline soaps can be associated with the contact with skin rashes.

The chemical components in the detergent can affect children quickly. It is mostly due their smooth skin which can't withstand high and extremely high concentrations of chemicals. It is crucial to protect your wellbeing of you and your loved ones members from the highly harmful soaps. It is much simpler to avoid the many problems which are in one form or another a result of soaps made from these substances by making your soap at home.

On the other side in the range, making soap at home can be extremely beneficial to your health. This is especially true if you choose to make use of an organic, natural and essential oils. You can make products that possess beneficial health properties. Furthermore it is possible to create soaps with particular purposes, such as soaps that serve antifungal or antiseptic soaps.

Glycerin is among the most important elements and an important moisture-trapping ingredient in the soap. But, the majority of commercial soap manufacturers eliminate the glycerin from their soaps and put it in their lotions and creams. Although it's an excellent idea however, it leaves you with a an "dry" bar that could be a better detergent for your car or laundry.

When you make soap, the selection of ingredients is inclusive or in this instance it is not removed, as opposed to commercial soaps. Dryness and irritation of the skin are the most common side effects with soap that is glycerin-free.

It's a good alternative

In our modern economic climate, everyone has the need for money that is left in our pockets...and everyone makes use of soap. Making soaps is a an incredibly low cost when in comparison to what you'd spend on the usual shampoo and soap for your body.

The soapmaking process can be done with a minimal cost. The entire process requires small expenditure. Did you even aware of this? Perhaps not, but I think. Many of you purchase soaps at stores, which can lead into spending more of money. Worst is that the products you purchase may cause harm for your skin. Since the disadvantages are evident, why would you buy soaps instead of making your soap at yourself? You will save lots of money and also most importantly, you will avoid allergic reactions that might happen. Additionally all of the ingredients that are natural and the equipment needed for soap making, such as soap molds are available at affordable prices.

It is possible to argue this way It is true that cheap soaps are affordable, they're true. But, if you're looking for high-quality soap, you'll have no choice but to pay higher for it. If you decide to buy the ingredients on a large scale and then making your soap in the batch, you'll definitely cut down on some of that cost. It is a given that a lot of components used to make soap like essential oils, can be used for a variety of uses and won't be thrown away when you've finished making your soap.

* Ideal for gift ideas

Virtually every boy as well as girl (come on and let us all know that it's the truth) like a nice smelling soap. If you create nice-smelling soaps, you'll not just be offering classy and personal items for you and your family as well, but you'll be able to distribute them with your loved ones as gifts.

In addition, it could be the perfect opportunity to introduce your family and friends acquaintances to the natural lifestyle. It is even more effective if you can describe the procedure, the ingredients, and the health benefits they could bring. If you can conversion to a sustainable lifestyle and your next venture arrives, you might have an extra pair of hands to help you complete the task.

When we talk about gifts, there's nothing better than pampering your most cherished friends and loved ones with gorgeous soaps. Your friends and family members will be stunned. It's not enough. Wait until they test it out! There will be a flurry of positive reviews and smiles everywhere I promise that you. They'll love the fragrance and it's good for their skin and will leave them feeling fresh after every bath. It's possible that your products may just trigger the waves of "it's amazing," particularly during those times of giving gifts.

* Fun and full of laughter

Making soap is a enjoyable and satisfying experience. There is nothing better than the satisfaction that comes from making something unique, beautiful and totally your own. It is a great way to connect with your loved ones

and the family members as well as family members during the process, with parents and daughters making memories with family and friends during the whole process.

This is where you can let your imagination run wild and, with a spark then you're set to go. Everybody, without second thought is going be able to benefit from your exquisitely created soaps. Something that been a hobby could turn into an obsession. Making new soaps to test your limits is a aspect of your knowledge in soapmaking.

* More than just cleaning.

Cleanliness is the primary reason for the development of soap. It is important to wash the dirt off while keeping your skin healthy while doing it. Another exciting aspect of making soap is the ability to add additional ingredients such as herbal supplements essential oils. It is easy to tailor the soap you make to meet your personal requirements for health, or just to boost the effectiveness of your aromatherapy during bathing. You can also include ingredients to exfoliate or other moisturizing agents to achieve greater outcomes.

Soap Making Equipment

The Scale

A scale is an essential piece of equipment needed to kick into your soap-making journey. Digital scales are the most effective and will read ounces, most often to the 1/10th of an ounce. The importance of measuring is that it guarantees you get the right chemical balance of soap precise. Scales are used to gauge everything, including your lye, liquids oil, and other the additions.

The Lye Container

When measuring the lye you'll need a transparent plastic measuring cupthat is specifically for the lye. It is best to mark it with "lye solely."

Lye is a poisonous chemical in its solid form. measurements you'll be taking throughout the process. It is essential that it be used just for this measurement only and for nothing other than that. A large measuring cup with capacity up to 12 ounces, dependent on the volume of batches you'll be creating is required.

The Mixing Vessel

The name implies that a mixing vessels are needed to mix oils and lye. This is carried out using a stainless steel container to stop the chemical reaction that can occur when mixing when mixing other metals. A stock pot is the most suitable option to make use of, which is around an 8-quart capacity, but it is all dependent on the size of the batch you're creating. The use of a stockpot permits you to work inside the pot, and prevent splashing the caustic lye substance just prior to saponification.

Safety

Security is a vital necessity in the soap manufacturing process, especially considering the chemicals used. For the highest level of security, make sure that you are wearing safety glasses to protect your eyes in the event there are any accidental splashes. As we mentioned previously the solution is dangerous before saponification and may cause significant damage and negative health consequences. Therefore, contact with eyes is not recommended at any time. Safety goggles are widely accessible and aren't as costly as they appear to be. They're available everywhere, at the majority of dollar stores or home improvement stores or even at the mass retail stores.

Spoon and Ladle

In the case of mixing or measuring and pouring like we mentioned earlier you'll require either stainless steel spoons or scoop made of stainless steel. Be sure to ensure that the items you use to mix are stainless steel to prevent any reactions with metal. You don't have to worry about it as these items can be easily found in local shops or in mass-wares stores.

Stick Blender

This single piece, along alongside the electronic scale is the most essential tool to make soap at home. While you may mix the mixture of lye and oils with your hands, the finished soap will be more smooth and harder to work with, but it will also be more professional if a stick mixer is used.

Mixing the ingredients, the stick blender will ensure that there is complete reflection of the ingredients until the final result is an efficient way, which ensures proper saponification and the best bars of soap. Stick blenders ' prices range from relatively cheap to excessively expensive. In the case of making soap, a basic stick blender will suffice.

Molds

Frames' uses for soap making can vary. Anything from dish washing tubs as well as silicone muffin cups to plastic storage containers as well as candy molds are all suitable for use. Additionally, you can be at the option of buying personalized soap mold on the internet or at the local craft shop. The choice is entirely yours to decide. But, we suggest to look for things that are squared off in the corners and over the round so that you don't waste time as well as the soap when trimming it to alter the shape of your soap bars.

It is also important to find molds that are able to be dismantled to expose the freestanding soap. Additionally, you could consider frames that are capable of being flexible to "pop" this soap upside down. It is best to avoid metal containers in this process and instead opt for the plastic that is soft or silicone.

Soap Making Techniques

Making your own soap at home is a blast and easy, as well as penny-wise innovative and satisfying. Nothing is more satisfying than taking an ounce of homemade soap to the bathroom or shower with you.

It does not matter if you're looking for an optimal choice of commercial soap, or simply seeking an adventure. Making soap is fun, and more than obsessive.

There are many different methods to make your soap. As long as you know the basic steps of soap making and you are ready to start today.

Here is a brief overview of the fundamental steps you can follow to create your own soap. This is a step-by-step tutorial through some fascinating soap-making tasks, that will provide you the details and the resources you need to begin making the soapy products you want to make.

The basic soap making methods.

Making soap is an arduous task when you don't have the right materials. If you're making soap in your home to serve a set of individuals, there are a variety of household items you could make use of. Pots, plastic juice jugs and milk cartons that have been abandoned as well as a sharp knife the thermometer, a whisk along with a container are a few things you can utilize to create soap. If, however, you're looking to begin a bigger scale business, such as an soap-making business and require financing for industrial soap-making equipment can allow you to save time and money.

How can this equipment be of assistance in the process of making soap? The first step is to must know the method you'd like to use for making your soap. Here are the methods that are used to make soap:

Chapter 2: Method Of Melting And Pouring

It's one of the most safe procedures. Melt as well as pour soap recipe could involve children , provided that they have safeguards against the hot splashes. There are no harmful chemicals, and the chances are low of injury, aside from minor burns. The process of melting and pouring is one of two choices to make soap that does not contain the use of lye.

Pour and melt bases are created in the process in advance. For soaps that are made to be crafty, purchase an uncut block from a wholesaler. Cut it using a strong knife, before melting it in an oven or microwave before adding the scent and color after pouring into molds. Once the soap is developed, it is removed from the mold and then it's all set to use. This soap-making method is quick and simple and requires approximately an hour or two to finish.

The advantage for melt-and-pour soaps are the level of security they provide when they're made. If not overheated the melting point never at a boil; in most cases the temperature isn't even enough to spark a scald, if you remove it from the source of heat the moment it has liquidized. Add-ins like fragrances and flower petals do not change as the soap is already neutral.

You can add anything you'd like like small toys, crushed herbs or even glitter. Soaps that melt and pour can be used with almost any mold unlike pure soaps that could melt molds, or react with aluminum.

Every thing has weaknesses, however. The most significant drawback of melt-and-pour soap is they're not completely "natural". Why? It is made up of a range of petroleum-based products.

A lot of people consider the soaps as drying, because they don't contain natural Glycerin (only added glycerin that is a manufactured item). The base is beautiful for crafting however, it's not the ideal choice for skin that is delicate.

If all you're looking for is a melt-and-pour soap study how to make a glycerin soap from scratch, and then build upon it. Everybody should be aware that this method of making soap requires the use of Lye. To make soap made of glycerin without lye you must use an already prepared base.

This is the simpler method since it is only buying already-made, unscented soap bases that are not colored or scented. Actually, you don't make the soap by hand just like you do with the cold process. When you use the melt and pour method however, you'll lose some control over your constituents. As a result your customization might be somewhat oriented toward the already-existing components of the bases of soap.

Below are the step-by-step instructions for this method:

Place soap in a microwave , and melt it at intervals of 10-25 seconds. It's all dependent upon the quantity of soap you wish to melt. 1 cup of chunks typically will take around 60 minutes (40 seconds, stirring before putting it back in the microwave for another 20 seconds) or in the microwave. Because microwaves differ in their capabilities, you must be vigilant about the soap you use. You don't want your soap to heat up too much. So, make sure to check the soap on a regular basis and give it an easy stir at each moment, and repeating the process until the lumps completely melt.

* Once the soap has melted then add it to the soap-safe fragrance oil (about 3/4-1 TBS per one pound of soap) Keep stirring until adding color. (Note that sometimes the fragrance oil

will cause soap to turn color. This is why I would recommend using the fragrance first, and then adding coloring). Also, you should do your best to not apply the fragrance oil if the soap is extremely hot, or else the fragrance oil could burn off. Allow the soap to cool to where you are able to put your finger inside it with no fear that you'll need to call paramedics later. But, it should not be cold enough that a skin layer begins to form on top. After adding your scent and dye, stir it gently until the additives are fully blended into the melted soap.

* With plenty of attention, pour your soap in clean molds. In my situation I would cover my molds using a layer made of petroleum jelly. It aids in the removal of soaps. It's now moment for you to "kill" these globules spraying the soap with alcohol. This is, however, an option. Personally, I like spraying into the globules(bubbles) and watch them disappear, though some are not fond using alcohol in soap. Relax the soap until it sets. If you're like me and are a bit agitated take it for up to 10 minutes. Then, carefully move the mold into an air-tight container until they're solid.

When your soap is firm and ready (usually within 30 hours to one hour) You can take them with care from the mold. They rarely pop out however, sometimes they're even more stubborn. If (rare however) they don't disappear after a gentle extraction, set them in the refrigerator for about half an hour (you might try freezing them as well) and then try to remove them again. You can make use of the soaps as soon when they are set.

Re-batching

French-pressed soaps are cold processed bars which have been ground repeatedly to form an even gel. They are then pressed into stunning shapes. Triple-milled soaps are grounded three times to increase the smoothness. This creates a luxurious feel and foam, but it also keeps the colors of the entire batch uniform. This means there's no streaking, and uneven shade of the resulting product. You shouldn't label these soaps to be "French-milled" in the absence of having them manufactured in France by this specific method of making soap; however, it is still possible to mill your soaps however.

By using existing cold-process soaps you can skip the steps that require the curing process and lye. Therefore, although milled soaps are less "from the ground" as cold or hot processed soaps but they can be made using the same organic ingredients.

Many soap makers create different soaps that make a "master" collection of cold-process soap to make a new batch (mill) to make top quality and chemically strong bars. Fragrances that would cause the soap that was originally made to turn copper-colored remain fresh after the process of re-batching. This soap-making technique is a great method to transform ugly soaping errors into appealing bars. If the soap that was created correctly made using exact ratios of lye to oil, but was separated during making, it could be mangled and then rebatched.

To re-batch, cut an ounce of soap made of cold processing. Mix it with a small amount of liquid, such as goat's milk. Soap must be allowed to melt slowly until it is stirred, and then quickly blends into the liquid. This can be accomplished in a jar, in a plastic bag with a heat-resistant seal set in boiling water, which may take up to an hour longer , or in using a microwave. When the mixture has melted to an extremely fluffy consistency and is ready to be added, you can add any additional ingredients, like the color or botanicals, and press it into molds. When it is cool and solidifies it's now ready for use.

Cold Process

The Cold Process used in soap making involves mixing of fixed oils (which comprise Coconut, Olive, and Palm) with an acid base (Sodium Hydroxide). Saponification is the outcome of the chemical process in which the oil's composition alters with the help of the lye in order to create an soap bar.

The most efficient soap making method for the professional soapmaker is the following method. Why? It's because in this process, the process of saponification is gradual, which means that crafters are given time to create stunning swirls and blends. The end product is typically more smooth than the hot process, however the product seizes (suddenly becomes hard). Many soap makers who's goal are to create a stunning product prefer the cold method over the hot method.

Its fluidity from the cold-process (CP) method permits you to make intricate swirls and patterns since the soap is infused with more fluid than those using the hot method.

The main benefit of this technique is that it is more appealing to the eye. The majority of heat is created through the chemical process and even though those temperatures may be as high as 180 degrees, or even melt other plastics there is no stirring in a the boiling point.

The cold process consists of these steps:
* Mixing lye and distillate water in one container , and getting the oils and fats to temperature in a separate container. Once the lye mix is cool, and the oil in a similar temp, the solution is gradually emptied into the oil.

The soap maker stirs the soap in a low or non-heat condition until it is at "trace." It could generally take anywhere from five minutes to around one hour maximum depending on the type of the oil that is that is used in the soap.

* After that, other ingredients like coloring or fragrance are added before the soap turns into heat-resistant non-metallic molds. The soap is kept in a warm location as it progresses through the gel phase of saponification. It's safe to make use of the soap within 24 to 48 hours, but it is much more supple and lasts longer if allowed to cure in an air-conditioned space for up to one-half months.

Since the mixture is in its alkaline state many hours, certain additives are not balanced. Flower petals do turn brown. The vanilla scent time to time transforms a white soap into a darker chocolate shade, except for when you are using stabilizer. Certain fruity or floral scents cause the soap becoming seize or ricing (when the soap's mixture is partially seizes into small clusters). If you are trained properly you will be able to solve each of these issues and create a fantastic soap in the final.

One of the biggest advantages of using a cold process for soap making is that it gives you complete oversight over all the components used in making up the composition of the soap.

Based on the ingredients you choose to use the process usually results in a strong bar of soap.

The drawback of the cold process is that there are security measures to be taken as well as the fact that some essential oils, fragrance oils and colorants can withstand the process of cooling, thus restricting the design options. In addition patience is an important quality since this process takes as long as a month of the curing process.

This method of soap making is labor-intensive. Why? because you start at "scratch" when you embark on your soap making journey, and the result is the result of all the work and effort put into obtaining the final product.

It is necessary to heat the oil you're planning to use up to around 100 degrees. Slowly and slowly add the lye water and let the mixture brew until it becomes thicker. Following that, add the desired scent and color. After that, pour the mixture into the molds, where it will sit for 24 hours before being frozen. Let the soap sit for an entire month to dry before it's ready for use.

Hot Process

With the same concentrations of lye and oil as in the cold process using the same concentrations of lye and oil, (HP) offers one major benefit over the cold process as the soap that results is ready to use almost immediately after the process is at an end. This is due to the fast-boiling temperatures create lye that could in the cold process require six weeks to soften.

People who make soap at home, and then use the hot process using double boilersand ovens or Crock pots. This is the most suitable soap making process for students in the soap making industry due to the flexibility with regards to the proportions of lye and oil, unlike the cold process, where the ratio is very precise.

All saponification takes place in the pot. It heats until the soap is at its "gel" state. Before chemically pure lye was readily available, soap makers from dowdy often utilized the hot soap making process since they were unable to secure the precise alkalinity level of the potash. So, they sat over the pots openly mixing and watching as the mixture was finished.

The Hot process includes these steps:
* Measurement of colorants and fragrances first, as there may not have enough time to add them in the final.
* Mix lye with liquid in the container and then pour the oil into a pan or crock pot. As opposed to cold processes the oils do not need to cool prior to mixing the lye.

It is then added to the lye mixture. is slowly added. Mix the soap till it is of the thickness of a pudding, referred to"trace. "trace."

*The soap is cooked at a moderate heat until it begins to bubble and then reaches the stage of gel.

* Following that is the addition of color , the soap maker then shovels the gooey, hot mix into the mold. After approximately forty-eight to eight hours the soap is removed then cut in the manner you prefer.

The soap made from Hot Process often doesn't look as stunning due to the fact that the process of saponification isn't as rapid as you would expect sometimes. The soap maker must be prepared to stir with color and fragrance before quickly putting it all in the form before it gets difficult. It's so hard that hot process soap tends to be uneven. Although it's not the most efficient method of making soap for soaps made by hand It's the method used to make washing soap that is later broken into smaller pieces that can be mixed with borax and wash soda.

Important note

There are a few points to be considered before deciding to utilize this method to make soap:

A considerable amount of time is required when using this method because you'll need to monitor the soap while it cooks. Thus, make sure you be prepared with a couple of hours reserved to take care of the soap you're planning to create. The good thing is that you'll be able do other things while the soap is cooking however, the downside is that it can keep you grounded until the point where you won't be able to leave your home. The process demands that you continuously monitor the soap's progress as it cooks.

It is evident that the appearance soap in a lot of cases tends to be a more rough and doesn't have as smooth a final as Cold process.

* Not all soap design concepts can be achieved using this method.

The distinction between cold and hot processes

As previously mentioned There are two main ways of making soap bar solid; they are the hot or cold process. The difference is that the cold process uses external heat, the saponification process as well as the curing time, and then the end that the soap.

External Heating and Saponification Period

Cold process soaps utilize the exothermic heat phenomenon that results by the acid and alkaline reactions of soap-making oils as well as the solution of lye.

In order to make soap using the cold process it is possible to reduce the solid oil's molasses to allow you to mix the extract of lye into the soap recipe's fat acids. There is no further heating in the actual saponification process. It can take about a day to the process to be completed.

To make soap by the hot process the external source of heat is utilized to speed up the process of saponification. The external source of heat could be an oven double boiler or Crock pot. The process of saponification is completed in about two hours.

Cure Time

Soaps that are made with the cold-process method can take between three and four weeks to create. Of course, it depends on where you reside. If, for instance are in a location with low humidity, such as Colorado the process may take soaps two weeks to dry. If you made the soaps using the hot process , one week of time for treatment is sufficient.

Aesthetics

Another distinction between the two methods is in how the soaps look. Cold process soaps appear to have an easier finish. Soaps that are made using heat process however have a more rougher surface. The difference occurs when you include the soap's additives.

In thermal process detergents you wait until the final minute time of "cook" period before adding ingredients. In Cold Process soaps, it is possible to put in the additives when your soap remains liquid , giving the soap a more smooth appearance.

Ingredients to make soap
There are many different ingredients that are available to make soap in your home. It could be a base, oil, fat, natural colorant, preservative or essential oils, each ingredient offers its own advantages when making soap. Each ingredient will give some or two distinctive features to the soap.
Before using any ingredient in soap made from natural ingredients it is crucial to be aware of the specifics of what ingredient it is and how it's likely to affect your final product.
Are you planning to learn just about one ingredient? It's not an issue. I've listed the ingredients and you could learn some things from the ones that appeal to those you love the most.

Chapter 3: The Base Oils Used To Make Soap

It's crucial to be aware that soap making processes work with any vegetable or animal oil or fat, but the soap making process is not possible with petroleum-based oils.

Traditional soaps were typically constructed using the most readily available oils and fats. Fats from animals, especially tallow and lard make excellent soaps.

With the advancement of global commerce over the past century or as a result, vegetable oils sourced in both the US and around the world have replaced a large portion of the lard and tallow that were once used for soap production particularly for soaps that were mass-produced.

The chemical composition of each different oil will have an effect on the final bar. For example, olive oil creates soap that is strong however, the bubbles are tiny and in some cases, thin. Coconut oil, however produces large, smooth chunks of granules. As a bar of soap. However, it may cause dryness to skin.

Handmade soap makers boast of the benefit of being able to create soaps that incorporate all kinds of specialty and primary oils to create their incredibly "perfect soap." Although it is likely to see the palm kernel and olive oils, coconut, or palm oils in the majority of soaps, you'll also find oils such as avocado, apricot and castor as well as almond, jojoba, hemp, and other oils from seeds or nuts or butters like mango Cocoa or Shea butter.

Handcrafted soap makers from all over the world are becoming more global aware, and therefore they are choosing their oils and ingredients not just for the superiority they provide to soap, but rather for their reliability and their fair trading practices.

N/B

It is crucial to keep in mind that the correct ingredients that make soap need to be added to allow saponification to happen. This chemical process it is the result of a chemical reaction that occurs between two bases and an acid, which produce salt. This will result in soap.

What ingredient in all natural soap can I choose to use to make the base? You may have asked the same question. I've too. I prefer to choose a chemical known as lye in soap making (sodium hydroxide). Although most soap makers adhere to this specific base, you can make soap using potassium hydroxide (potash) as the base.

Lye can produce a stronger and thicker bar of soap whereas potash makes a comfortable and softer soap bar. Actually, I'd consider using potash as a base for making liquid soaps.

The soapmaking process requires acid.

I am sure you will agree that picking your base does not give you the space to experiment with your ideas. One of the most enjoyable aspects of making soap is that you are able to create a variety of kinds of soap by altering your base's acid and reacting with it. The change in the soap recipe causes the soap to change into its own distinct shape.

Here's a list of acids you could think of using when making soap:

* Avocado oil
* Coconut oil
* Castor oil
* Cottonseed oil
* Olive oil
* Palm oil
* Peanut oil
*Soybean oil (vegetable shortening)
* Oil sweet almond
* Jojoba oil
* Kukui nut oil
* Shea Butter
*Tallow (beef)
* Lard

The choice of one method over the other is an individual decision. None of the methods makes any solvent technique superior to the other.

The water ingredient is a key component.

Is water a component? Yes, it is and can be used to create the lye solution that is mixed together with oils. The amount of water is determined by the soap recipe. But, it should be enough to allow the oil and lye molecules to form soap. The bulk of the water will evaporate from the soap as it dries over time.

Perfume ingredients

Although some soaps made by hand don't contain any aroma-enhancing ingredients The majority are made of essential oils made from plants and fragrance oils based on the soap maker's preferences and the market need.

Plant-extracted Essential Oils

Like the name implies, essential oils are derived in plants, and they have the quality of being "natural." There are many ways of getting essential oils however the variety of possible scents is not enough. The soap makers and perfumers with experience mixing essential oils are able to create stunning scents by using only essential oils. Certain essential oils are expensive, and therefore are not suitable to incorporate them into soaps made of pure ingredients. The real rose essential oil for instance, needs approximately 6,000 tons of petals in order to make around 16 oz and can fetch up to $4,000.

Fragrance Oils

Fragrance oils are derived in the form of aromatic chemicals, which are then recombined to create the scents we recognize and love.

In certain instances, fragrance oils blends could contain essential oils as well as "indistinguishable natural compounds" (compounds produced in a laboratory , but having the same molecular structure like those found that are found in the natural world).

The majority of food-like scents (i.e. chocolate, butter, coffee) and fruit-based scents (i.e. blackberry, mango, apple and cucumber) are synthetic aroma oils. Soap that is perfumed with real flowers like lilac jasmine or rose, is created using aroma oils because the oils from these flowers are difficult or expensive to make.

Coloring ingredients

The dyes are the coloring agents. But, they must get approval from the Food and Drug Administration (FDA) before they can be used in soaps of any kind. Mica is a good example, and is commonly used to alter the color of soap.

Any ingredient used in a soap or makeup with the aim of changing the color must be on the list of Food and Drug Administration-approved colorants and suitable for that particular purpose. This is due to the serious negative effects certain colorants could cause to the skin.

For example, certain coloring agents are not suitable for use on the lips as are others that aren't suitable to be used in products for the eye.

Alongside color additives certain ingredients can change the color of soap. One example is the addition of French green clay into soap. The soap will change to the color of green. Cinnamon however will make the soap brown, and paprika orange. Do not confuse these ingredients with altering the color of soap. They possess other properties that they add into the finished product.

Preservative Agents

One issue that is faced by soap makers when using naturally-sourced ingredients is they will degrade faster than those made with synthetic ingredients. In an effort to stop this problem the soap makers add preservatives into the soap.

I strongly support making use of organic preservatives that are natural. Beware of the synthetic forms of prophylaxes (preservatives). In the end, if you were initially tempted to go with unnatural prophylaxes you could use ingredients for soapmaking that will eliminate the need for treatment. Good point you think?

Please note that you don't necessarily have to include an ingredient to preserve your soap. In the majority of cases, it depends on the oil used and the time you intend to store your final product.

Here's a listing of some naturally-derived preservatives often utilized in soaps, when the need is for them:

* Grapefruit seed extract
* Tocopherols
* Root oil from carrots

There are two other ingredients for soap making that soap makers often incorporate in their final product Colorants, and Essential oils/fragrances.

Pure cleansersmade of oils, lye, and water, don't require preservatives. There aren't many prophylaxes in hand-crafted soap. Some liquid soapsthat contain high percentages of water, might require chemical treatments. The soap bases that are ready-made might contain preservatives or may require them.

Nutrients Essential Natural Skin Care Ingredients

The two ingredients that make soap (acid as well as base) are, theoretically speaking, the only ingredients that are required for soap making. But are you looking to appear boring? Absolutely not!

Here's a list with ingredients I've used in the past, and will keep using often to make my

soaps have that extra look and add a touch of my personal style:
* Aloe Vera
* Balsam copaiba
* Honey
* Oatmeal is an excellent ingredient in natural soap
* Alfalfa meal
* Seaweed

Recipes for soap
The skin of those who are sensitive to soaps are usually susceptible to scent oils, and therefore they are often left out of soap making for skin that is sensitive.
Use the basic soap-making procedures This batch, especially when you don't use any scents or colorants is relatively simple.
Gentle Hemp And Shea Soap Recipe
Ingredients:
* 10 percent Shea Butter
*30% beef tallow, or lard
* Coconut oil is 25% of the total.
* Castor oil 5%
* 17 percent hemp seed oil
* 13% olive oil
* 3 tbsp. white clay.
* 1/2 tsp. Titanium dioxide, dispersed into 1 teaspoon. Olive oil

* 1 tbsp. hemp hearts
Method
Make use of the traditional cold method to make this soap. Pour the soap batter into an container and allow it to mark using the help of a stick blender. Take a quarter of the dough and place it in another bowl. It will create the transparent middle layer. Incorporate titanium oxide to the mix and stir until it becomes a lighter shade. Place half of the dark green in your mold. followed by the lighter layer, then the remainder portion of the thicker layer. smooth it out as well that you are able to. Allow the batter to set for around 20 minutes before you add the hemp heart over the batter. Allow the soap to set for around a month, it is then yours to utilize it for cleaning.

Honey and Milk Soap Recipe
Ingredients:
* 1 lb. The Soap Base of Goat's Milk
* 3 tbsp. Organic Raw Honey
* Soap with Red and Yellow Colorant (optional)
Method
Cut your soap's base in cubes put them into an measuring cup. The base should be microwaved for around 20-30 seconds in increments, while stirring each time. This is to ensure that the base is well melted. Mix in the honey organic and a few drops the colorant. Pour the soap

that has been liquefied into the mold and let it cool for anywhere between 30 minutes and two hours. Then , remove the soap out of the mold.

Sea Mud Soap Recipe

Sea mud, which is referred to in the form of French clay, has substances that are beneficial to the skin since they are able to be used for cleansing and nourishing.

Ingredients:

* 20 oz. olive oil
* 10 oz. coconut oil
* 11.4 oz. distillated water
* 4.2 oz. Lye
* 2-4 level tablespoons of sea mud
* 1/2 ounce essential oils

Method

Make use of the hot process for creating soap using this instance. Make sure you add essential oils after the soap mixture has cool slightly, otherwise they'll lose their scent. The soap should be left for 2 to 3 weeks for all the properties of conditioning to set.

Pure Coconut Oil Recipe

Ingredients:

* 33 oz. coconut oil. degrees
* 4.83 ounces lye
* 12.54 oz. water
* .5 - 1 ounce essential oils (optional)

Method

Follow the standard hot process procedure and allow the soap to sit for 2 weeks to allow the conditioning properties to fully cure.

Although other bars need around 24 hours to cut and cut, coconut oil creates an extremely tough bar that requires cutting when it's sufficiently hard.

Thyme and Witch Hazel Facial Bar Recipe

Ingredients:

* 1/2 cup freshly chopped or 1/4 cup dried Thyme
* 8 oz. The Simmering Distilled Warm Water
* 15 oz. Olive Oil
* 8 oz. Coconut Oil
* 4 oz. Sunflower Oil
* 2 oz. Castor Oil
* 1 oz. Tamanu Oil
* 4.17 oz. Sodium Hydroxide Lye
* 0.5 oz. Raw Honey
* 1 oz. Witch Hazel

Method

Prepare the thyme-infused water. Place the fresh thyme inside an oven-proof jar. Pour the boiling hot distilled liquid and let it sit until it cools. Strain and set aside. If you are using dry thyme, you must steep it for 30 minutes , or the water will become too dark and cause discoloration of the soap. Blend the hazel with honey, and then set aside. Gradually add the lye mixture to the thyme solution after it is fully cooled. slowly stir it until the lye has completely dissolved.

The remainder of the recipe is stated in the cold procedure and the soap is left to cure for between four and six weeks.

Create Your Own Scrubs It's too easy not to!

A lot of people aren't thinking about making their own products even though gardening is a favorite pastime for the majority of people. Growing your own herbs and fruits will not only help you save money , but also help to live a healthier life. The homemade scrubs and soaps are similar and you will be able to know the products you're using for your face. Plus, you will be able to regulate it and save money over the long term!

There are many good advantages to making your own body scrubs and soaps. A scrub for your body and face made at home will be more organic because you've already identified the ingredients you're making use of. A lot of people buy cosmetics that come with lengthy, long lists of strange ingredients. If we make the effort to look up these ingredients, we realize that we would never wish to even a tenth of those chemical compounds on our skin. Certain people may prefer an organic or natural product but they are expensive.

What's the solution? Making your own, of course.

An homemade scrub for your body may be a great present! The gift is customizable for your loved ones according to the individual preferences of each person and the holiday you're celebrating, as well as any allergies they may suffer from. It is what you think about that matters, and the present of homemade scrubs is sure to have plenty of thought with it.

If you make your own soaps and scrubs you can customize them to your liking. Whatever scent you decide to use is yours to make. If you are a fan of peppermint, you can definitely create the perfect face scrub using peppermint. have a Christmas celebration in July! Scrubs aren't just natural, however their flexibility can make them quite fun too.

We discussed the toxins used in the majority of cosmetics these days. They can cause those with the highest levels of sensitivities experience adverse reactions, such as irritation, redness and worsening skin problems. Making a homemade scrub instead of buying an expensive cream that has an ingredient list from the grocery store can be beneficial for sensitive skin. A lot of scrubs you can find in stores have those frightful mysterious ingredients and can be dangerous and irritating to skin that is sensitive. This is particularly true for people suffering from ailments like rosacea, psoriasis or eczema.

Organic, natural products, whether they are customizable or organic even though we might require them due to sensitive skin, or for any other reason, they come with an expensive price. The organic food stores in your area can supply you with the pure and natural products for your beauty needs however, their cost is enough to make you weak. What is the solution? It's not as if you could change the way you react to your skin! The best way to save hundreds of dollars on natural creams is to create your own! Scrubs are simple for you to create at-home, and they are so versatile, you'll be amazed to discover that you have the majority of those ingredients in your kitchen cupboard.

What's cooking in your kitchen? Scrubs are so simple and simple - so why don't you start making one now? Since, in truth one of the most compelling reasons to create one yourself is due to the simplicity of the procedure!

The best part is that it isn't difficult to accomplish. A little effort and investment in the ingredients, and you could prepare a month's supply in just a few hours. It's worth the effort. In this article we go over the many advantages that you can get from creating your own facial scrubs, and what kind of skin will shine when you make use of the natural ingredients you can make at home.

This guide offers tips on what equipment you'll require and which ingredients are the best to start with, and delve into the types of skin and which ingredients work best for you. It's time to begin creating your own body and face scrubs!

Making an Scrub
Equipment

As you can see, salt and sugar scrubs are very simple to create and can prove effective when used regularly. If, however, you're new to the DIY cosmetics it is possible that you are unaware that the ingredients to make your next facial scrub exfoliating are at hand in the kitchen.

Fortunately, it's easy to create the sugar scrub of your dreams. If you are aware of the right tools to use and the right tools, you can create your own scrubs each week. A lot of the ingredients often used to make sugar scrubs at home are available in your kitchen regularly. One of the advantages of making your sugar scrub from scratch is the wide range of ingredients.

If you're planning to for your personal scrubs you should choose an old container to use for storage. An option that is popular is a glass jar, like the sauce or jam glass bottle, a jam or sauce jar or mason Jar. Create

Be sure to use an appropriate lid and seal in the event that you have leftovers and wish to use it in the next week (use it in a hurry, especially in the event that you've had food!).

To make the scrub, prepare an enormous mixing bowl and spoon, and then gather all the ingredients. Mix the ingredients according with the recipes, then ensure that all ingredients mix well. It's fairly simple because most recipes make use of oil, which is a wonderful unifier! Mix thoroughly before applying the scrub on your body and face.

You can keep your homemade scrub in however you want and especially when you're creating something unique and giving it out as a present. You can use ribbon or a personalized label to embellish the exterior of the jar or container, and make it truly your personal.

The appeal of DIY facial scrubs lies in their flexibility, convenience and the frequency with which we discover the ingredients within our homes. This is true for the techniques and storage too.

Basic Techniques

If there's going to be one thing that will frequently mentioned throughout this tutorial is that the process of making an easy scrub at home is not difficult. Therefore, naturally the methods used are simple to follow. It's as if everyone could master it!

The process of creating the Scrub

It is the first thing to make scrub. Mix all the ingredients the ingredients in the bowl (or follow any directions that might differ) and prepare to truly revitalize your skin. After your scrub is applied happens when all the magic occurs. Be sure you put your hair in a ponytail prior to applying the scrub, unless happy with baking soda in your hair. Many people aren't. But this is your time to pamper yourself!

Before Utilization

The most crucial tool is required, always cleanse your face prior to washing it. It is the most efficient way to wash your face using warm water. This will unblock your pores and allow you to cleanse your face of oils and dirt. You can also do this by putting the warm, wet towel over your face.

By using the Scrub

If you've applied the scrub on your skin, ideal tools to use is the scrub brush or loofah. It is important not to go overboard and you're trying to effectively exfoliate your skin. A facial loofah or sponge or brush are fantastic instruments to maximize the exfoliation from DIY facial scrubs.

Then, rinse your face with warm water just like you would using any other cleansing product or masque. Spray cold water onto your skin to reduce pores and prevent fresh dirt and oil from getting into areas where it isn't needed.

If you've created an amazing facial scrub and have a bit left over, save it to use later within an airtight container. You will have to apply it within a few days, particularly if are using ingredients that are food grade like oatmeal, bananas and almond oil.

It is suggested that you apply a facial scrub once to two times a week. However, people who have sensitive skin must be mindful whenever using facial cleanser. Be attentive to your skin and when it starts to feel irritated or red, change the frequency of your use or scrubs.

Ingredients, Oils and herbs
In the middle of every refreshing and natural home-made scrub is the components. The ingredients must be natural or organic. If you're

using food grade ingredients that means they are all-natural ingredients. As a healthy lifestyle suggests, using top quality cosmetic products requires you to be aware of the ingredients and comprehend the ingredients you're putting on your skin.

There are some essential ingredients that are used within homemade recipe for homemade scrubs. They are easily accessible and are much less expensive than pre-made scrubs that are sold in the stores. Most of the time, you'll have a variety of ingredients in your kitchen and you may not even know that you've got them.

Sugar

Many people struggle to eliminate sugar out of their diets however it's not easy because sugar is addictive and can lead to the accumulation of excess body fat. But , don't be worried that a bit of sugar will never harms anyone, whether both inside and out - but and not on the outside!

Sugar can be surprisingly beneficial to your skin, which makes it one of the two main ingredients of a homemade scrub.

It is an organic humectant which is a chemical which absorbs moisture from the environment and then into your skin. Sugar makes a wonderful base for moisturizing a face mask, and also helps to keep it inside. Also, it contains glycolic acid that is an alpha-hydroxy acid (or

AHA). It can help to increase the lifespan that your cells in the skin, and create a more youthful-looking skin i.e. younger looking skin. It also helps treat sun-damaged skin and has anti-aging properties. It is also, of course it's an excellent exfoliant. The exfoliating power of this ingredient makes your skin feel refreshed soft and soft.

Scrubs make use of white sugar as well as granulated according to what you have available or the flavor you like. For recipes like vanilla scrubs or coffee scrubs the brown sugar will be more pleasing to the eye. Overall making use of sugar for your scrubs can be an overall enjoyable experience. It's a pleasant scent as well. Your skin is sure to be grateful to for it.

Salt

Sugar scrubs aren't the most delicious scrubs, salt is the 2nd essential ingredient in scrubs. The majority of people prefer sea salt, however there are some who use iodine that we utilize in the kitchen because of its accessibility. However, sea salt contains many important minerals that we require: sodium magnesium, calcium, as well as potassium.

These minerals are crucial in the development and maintenance of our skin all the way to its cell communication. Without these essential elements our skin may appear dried, dull inflamed and even flaky. This is not a good indicator of the overall health of our skin.

Utilizing salt in masks and facial scrubs it is possible to benefit from sea salt's anti-inflammatory properties. It also helps regulate the production of oil in your skin and help retain the moisture is required to keep it looking radiant.

Salt really does aid in achieving the perfect balance. But, if you do use salt for a scrub, it's best to ensure it's finely crushed so that you don't the most pleasant revitalization, but an irritable and painful one instead.

Salt can also be used for other reasons in your routine of beauty. It can be utilized in your hair to fight hair dandruff, and also to stimulate positive growth of your scalp. If it is added to the warm bath, salt aids in cleanse the pores. It is also employed as a tooth whitener together with baking soda.

Oils

Natural oils aren't the most secret beauty secrets - they've always come in the bag when it comes to this fantastic moisturizer. We all benefit from the power of oils such like coconut oil and olive oil. If we are enthralled by oils to beautify, it's heard from the top of the mountain. This is probably why oils are among the most essential ingredients to make your own scrub.

Fortunately, the oil you select to use for your facial scrub can alter based on your personal preference sensitive skin, any allergies you might suffer from. Make sure to use products that are suitable on your face. Remember homemade scrubs are designed to improve your skin So any harmful ingredients are not to be included in the mixture.

Oils are crucial in a scrub since they're intended to rid your skin of dead skin cells and leave your skin feeling soft and hydrated. Oils offer a natural moisturizing effect to your skin. They is used in a manner that won't cause breakouts on the skin, or trigger irritation. We recommend that you apply them with care, it is important to not use an oil that is too heavy for skin with acne or that is too strong of an irritant for sensitive skin. Also, be sure to understand your skin's needs before applying anything to it. For oils, you can use food grade or not insofar that it's suitable for skin, and is a complete food item.

There are numerous oils you can choose from when making your own scrub or if you just want an all-natural lotion for the skin.

There are however four main name brands within the beauty industry including avocado oil, argan oil, coconut oil along with olive oil.

Argan Oil.

Argan oil is now an effective and popular cosmetic product, and has amazing scent to match.

It's rich in omega-3 fatty acids as well as vitamin E, which are linked with healthier, more youthful skin. When applied correctly to your skin argan oil

A lot of people also believe in the use of Moroccan oil for treating damaged and dry hair. The range of products from shampoos to conditioner as well as hair masks and the hair mousse we desire argan oil that will nourish our hair to the roots! Its scent is exquisite and always a plus.

Avocado Oil.

It's more than just the perfect dip for your party Avocado oil can help you for those who suffer from dry and sensitive skin. As with Argan oil is rich in vitamins E as well as omega-3 fats that aid in cell function. People who suffer from sensitive skin conditions such as psoriasis , can experience a reduction in the redness and inflammation that is typically caused by skin issues.

It's more than just beauty. taking avocado oil in the form of a drink can lower blood pressure and to prevent bone loss that benefits the joints of your teeth and your jaw.

Do you not love it oils that have so many wonderful uses? This is why essential oils have become more popular in bathrooms and kitchens.

Coconut Oil.

It is impossible to go anywhere without being surrounded by coconut oil. It is extremely popular nowadays and is a great thing. Coconut oil can be costly at some health food stores but since it's becoming more commonplace you can buy it in many stores for 10 or less.

While you can pick an oil from coconut that does not smell the sweet scent of this oil is a favourite for many. Coconut oil is great for those who have extremely sensitive skin or Eczema. A lot of people also use coconut oil to revive damaged hair or dry hair. It is also eaten or added to toothpastes that whiten teeth. It's impossible to fail by purchasing a huge coconut oil container and having a blast with it.

Olive Oil.

It's not a bad idea to walk straight into the kitchen to apply the usual olive oil that is extra-virgin on your hair or face. It is an all-natural moisturizer that any beauty enthusiast should use. Although it is not known to cause allergies but it is heavier than the majority of oils. Those who are prone to acne shouldn't make use of olive oil. It is a great option to reduce the appearance of acne for certain, but only when used in moderation, as it's heavier than other oils listed on this list. Oil can destroy oil, but olive oil is more potent than the rest. It is, naturally an excellent moisturizer as well as remover of makeup.

Olive oil is also used in leave-in and shampoo conditioners in addition to face masks and hair masks (but you can create your own, it's far more organic!). Also, it leaves a pleasant smell to your hair with only a few sprays.

Chapter 4: Essential Oils

Essential oils can also be important in making homemade scrub. Essential oils are fragrant and adaptable, and are typically sourced in plants. It comes from the leaf, flower or bark, root branch or seed from the plants. It is amazing that there are hundreds of these essential oils. They give your scrub different scents which means you can choose the right one for what you're feeling (promotion of calm or wakefulness) or pick the most appealing scent to use as an energy boost.

There are three methods to make use of your favourite essential oils. A lot of people prefer to sit and relax with the scent of tea tree, lavender or peppermint. It's inevitable when you add 5-10 drops of essential oils that is common to your salt or sugar scrub. Diffusion utilizes diffusers, vaporizers, sprays or mists to fill a space or area with a stimulating or soothing smell.

What essential oils should you select to help lift or improve your mood? The most popular scents for relaxing are lavender, frankincense, and spearmint. If you want to feel as if you're being awake, you can try peppermint, a citrus scent like tangerine or orange as well as rosemary or basil. The use of scents to boost moods or mental state is called aromatherapy and is extremely beneficial for many. This could be directly applied to the application of essential oils for body scrubs.

Scrubs are an approach that is topical to essential oil application. Scrubs, lotionsand body mists, facial creams and massage oil are just a few ways for applying topical oils. It is recommended to dilute your essential oils as the concentration is so high that just few drops are needed to get the product you apply to your skin.

Take care not to consume essential oils or apply them for cooking, and avoid applying essential oils that are not dilute on your skin since they may be harmful, depending on the oil.

Fresh Herbs

The usage for fresh herb is similar to using essential oils, whether you're making use of sage to enhance the smell or for its healing properties. Dry the herbs to crush and then put them in an homemade scrub like the other ingredients. Similar to essential oils these herbs are linked to aromatherapy and positive mood changes.

The natural ingredients are extremely adaptable and will not just provide your skin with moisture, but also keep it healthy with only natural ingredients. If you eliminate those long-winded mysterious ingredients, you allow your skin glow.

Scrub Recipes
The skin that is sensitive can appear in many kinds. As mentioned in the homemade scrubs made specifically designed for skin that is dry, issues such as eczema or rosacea can also trigger sensitive skin. Certain people are born with sensitive skin than normal, so they should use natural solutions to clean clothing, moisturize their skin, and also wash. It could be a test.

There are some things to consider when suffering with sensitive skin, meaning you shouldn't suffer any more.

Avoid chemicals and long-winded substances

Products sold over-the-counter can have adverse reactions in people who have sensitive skin. Chemicals and fragrances can trigger reactions like pustules, bumps and erosion. The ingredients you have to Google and then seek your Ph.D to comprehend isn't suitable for those with sensitive skin. Beware of products that are advertised for normal skin.

Dry skin isn't your friend

Dry skin is not able to protect the nerve endings of the skin. In addition, sensitive skin may also flush quite quickly. When conditions like allergic contact dermatitis can cause dry, dried skin, it can also result in skin injuries exposed to excessive sunlight, cold or other harsh surroundings. For those suffering from sensitive skin and allergies it's not always easy to find a product to moisturise with.

Fortunately, You Can DIY

There are a variety of treatments and lotions - which are better for those suffering from these issues ranging from moderate to severe that cause skin sensitivity. However, there are many who have problems with these drugs and creams because they contain chemicals that may not suit everyone's individual skin. Many people opt for natural options like oil-based lotions, homemade products, as well as DIY body salt or sugar scrubs.

There are numerous advantages that natural ingredients provide to sensitive skin. There aren't any lab-created chemicals and only foods that you know about. Additionally, many who suffer from sensitive skin are forced to resort to costly soaps and creams, which puts an expensive price on the need. If you make your scrubs at home and soaps, you are not only can use them several times per week , but they're made of ingredients are already within your home. Be cautious not to scrub too hard because it can alter the benefits of these ingredients that improve skin.

The ingredients for dry skin

Coconut Oil: The coconut oil is able to accomplish what many oils can help moisturize and protect the skin from the elements that cause irritation and dryness. It's recommended for those who have dry and sensitive skin and it rarely triggers breakouts or allergies.

Vitamin E Vitamin E is the ideal blend of antioxidants, which help improve the skin's defenses from environmental irritants and elements. Make sure you are using facial cleanser that is sensitive with vitamin E or use some drops of vitamin E in every scrub.

Oatmeal: Oatmeal has always been a mighty ingredient in aiding in the reduction of inflammation caused by irritation of the skin, rashes, and is a mother's answer to chickenpox. When it's ground into a fine powder, it can be utilized as a facial cream or scrub. It is a good source of anti-histamines Oats help soothe irritation and also protect skin.

The natural ingredients in this blend will not just calm your skin, but also ensure that they have the protection they require to be calm and calm when dealing with elements and ingredients which aren't gentle.

Tropical Facial Scrub

Ingredients:
* 1/4 cup pureed pineapple
* 1/4 cup pureed papaya
2. 2 Tablespoons Brown Sugar
1. 1 Tablespoon almond oil
Honey 1 teaspoon
Method
A facial scrub made of two vibrant and tropical fruits is an essential for the spring and summer months. The summer months are the most sunny of the year leave a lot of us craving refreshing and sweet fruit like papaya and pineapple. The unique scent will take you out of your house and into the ocean within a matter of seconds.

Kiwi Sugar Scrub
Ingredients:
1 cup of white sugar
* 3 tablespoons safflower oils
* 1 kiwi, mashed
Method
Although this is a straightforward dish, the use of safflower oil may be extremely beneficial. Safflower oil has linoleic acids that can clear pores and stimulate new cell growth in the skin. Some even claim that it makes you appear younger. Remember, oil destroys oil!

Raspberry Lip Scrub
Ingredients:

* 3 raspberries that are perfectly ripe
White sugar, 6 tablespoons
2 Tablespoons Coconut Oil
Method
Are you in need of a refreshing and rejuvenating scrub? This raspberry-scented delight will bring you back to peace after a tiring day.

Sweet Tomato Scrub
Ingredients:
* 1 tomato cut in half
* 1 teaspoon sugar
Method
This scrub is very simple. Simply cut the tomato into half and sprinkle the sugar inside. Make use of each tomato half to gently scrub your body or face should you wish to use.

Tomatoes are gentle on skin. If you've had skin damaged by sun exposure and you are looking forward to the high level of lycopene found in tomatoes which will shield you from sun damage.

The spiced Apple Cider Sugar Scrub
Ingredients:
* 1 Cup Brown Sugar
1 cup Coconut Oil
* 1/2 teaspoon cinnamon
* 10-15 drops Apple Cider Essential Oil
* 4 drops Orange Essential Oil

Method

A different recipe that is seasonal This scrub is sure to allow you to escape from a sleepy night and enjoy an enjoyable fall afternoon at the parks. Spice and apple cider are two scents that will bring many of us home for Thanksgiving and Halloween These types of scents can be extremely therapeutic.

Chapter 5: Lotions And Creams For Dry Skin

Recipes for lotions

Chamomile Cashmere Lotion

Ingredients:

7.8 ounces water distilled

* 1 ounce coconut oil

* 1 ounce olive oil

* 2 ounces beeswax

• 1 teaspoon vitamin E oil

*1 teaspoon shea butter

*20 drops essential oil of chamomile

Method

1. A bowl is used to mix the distilled water with Vitamin E oil.

2. Pour butter, beeswax as well as oil, into a double boiler , and stir.

3. After melting completely, place the wax and oil mix into the food processor , and let it cool. (about 20 minutes)

4. Once the oil mixture has become cool but not hard make sure to turn the food processor off low, and slowly add the water.

5. When the lotion is smooth, you can include the essential oils.

6. After another 15 minutes, transfer the lotion into the pump dispenser.

7. Place in the refrigerator, and take pleasure in it!

This lotion is great for skin that is sensitive. Shea butter, the oils and chamomile essential oils are the most important and effective ingredients in this recipe that helps sensitive skin. The recipe can be stored in the fridge for up to 2 weeks.

Mosquito Bite Relief Lotion

Ingredients:

* 7 ounces aloe vera gel
* 2 ounces coconut oil
2 ounces of beeswax
15 drops essential oil of basil
Five drops tea tree essential oil

Method

1. Pour butter, beeswax along with oil in a double-boiler and stir.

2. When the wax is completely melted, pour the wax and oil mix into the food processor , and allow to cool. (about 20 minutes)

3. Once the oil mixture has become cool, but still soft then turn the food processor off low, and slowly add the water.

4. Once the lotion has become smooth, include the essential oils.

5. After another few minutes, put the lotion into the pump dispenser.

6. Keep in the refrigerator and have fun!

This lotion is ideal for those with sensitive skin as well as the relief of mosquito bites. Aloe Vera and coconut oil and the essential oil blend are the primary and active ingredients that make up this recipe. Basil essential oil can help alleviate the itching mosquito bites. Keep it in the refrigerator for up to two weeks.

Rose Face Toner Lotion

Ingredients:

* 7 Ounces of rose water
* 2 ounces coconut oil
* 1 teaspoon of beeswax
• 1 teaspoon vitamin E oil
* 5 drops essential rose oil
*5 drops Geranium oil

Method

1. In a bowl, mix distilled water and the vitamin E oil.

2. Put oil and beeswax in an oven double boiler. Stir.

3. After melting completely, place the wax and oil mix in the food processor and allow to cool. (about 20 minutes)

4. Once the oil mixture has become cool but still soft switch the food processor to low, and slowly add the water.

5. Once the lotion has become smooth, you can add essential oils.

6. After another few minutes, put the lotion into the pump dispenser.

7. Place in a fridge and take pleasure in it!

This lotion is suitable for skin that is sensitive. Coconut oil, rose water and essential oils are the primary and active ingredients that make up this recipe. Rose water and essential oil can be beneficial to people with sensitive skin. Keep them in the refrigerator for up 2 weeks.

Honeybee Lotion

Ingredients:

* 6 8 ounces of distilled water
* 1 teaspoon of neroli water

2 ounces of coconut oil

* 1.5 grams of beeswax
* 1 ounce of honey that is raw

1. 1 tablespoon of Vitamin E oil

1 teaspoon Shea butter

2. Drops of essential oil

2. Drops of essential oil of chamomile

2. Drops of essential lavender oil

Method

1. In a bowl, mix the distilled water and the vitamin E oil.

2. Pour honey, beeswax, shea butter, and oil into a double-boiler on low heat. Stir.

3. After melting is complete, pour the wax and oil mix in the food processor and allow to cool.

4. When the oil mixture is cool, but not completely soft, switch the food processor off low, and slowly add the water.

5. When the lotion is smooth, add essential oils.

6. After another few minutes, put the lotion into the pump dispenser.

7. Place in the refrigerator, and take pleasure in it!

This lotion is great for skin that is sensitive. The most active and effective ingredients in this recipe include vital oils. They are neroli water coconut oil , and shea butter. This mix is perfect for people who have skin sensitivities. It can be stored in the fridge for up to two weeks. Do not make this recipe if are allergic to honey.

Baby's Touch Lotion

Ingredients:

* 6 six ounces of water distilled
* 1 teaspoon of neroli water
* 2 1 ounces of oil from rice bran
1 tablespoon of Jojoba butter
*1 1/2 ounces beeswax
1. 1 tablespoon of Vitamin E oil
Three drops essential lavender oil
* 2 drops of essential rose oil

Method

1. A bowl is used to mix the water that has been distilled and the Vitamin E oil.

2. Pour butter, beeswax along with oil in a double-boiler and stir.

3. After melting completely, place the wax and oil mix in the food processor and allow to cool. (about 20 minutes)

4. When the oil mixture is cool but not hard make sure to switch the food processor to low, and slowly add the water.

5. Once the lotion has become smooth, you can include the essential oils.

6. After another few minutes, put the lotion into an empty pump dispenser.

7. Place in a fridge and have fun!

This lotion is great for those with sensitive skin. The essential oil mix, jojoba oil, along with rice bran oil, are the main and principal ingredients that make up this recipe. Keep it in the refrigerator for up to two weeks.

Cotton Cloud Lotion

Ingredients:

* 4 four ounces of distilled water
* 3 three ounces of water containing neroli
* 1 tablespoons of almond sweet oil
* 1 ounce olive oil
* 2 pounds of beeswax

1. 1 tablespoon of Vitamin E oil

Five drops essential lavender oil

*3 drops essential oil of chamomile

2. Drops of essential oils of sandalwood

Method

1. A bowl is used to mix the water that has been distilled and the Vitamin E oil.

2. Pour the oil and beeswax into an oven double boiler. Stir.

3. After melting is complete, pour the wax and oil mix in the food processor and allow to cool.

4. When the oil mixture is cool, but still soft then switch the food processor off low, and slowly add the water.

5. Once the lotion has become smooth, you can include the essential oils.

6. After another 15 minutes, transfer the lotion into an empty pump dispenser.

7. Keep in the refrigerator and have fun!

This lotion is suitable for those with sensitive skin. The essential oils as well as Sweet almond oil comprise the major ingredients that make up the formulation. Sweet almond oil is great for people with sensitive skin. It can be stored in the fridge for up to two weeks.

Rose Garden Lotion

Ingredients:

* 8 Ounces of rose water
* 2 tablespoons coconut oil
* 2 teaspoons of oil sweetened with almonds
* 1 ounce of cornstarch
* 1 an ounce of beeswax
* Five drops Geranium essential oil

* Five drops essential lavender oil
Method

1. Put cornstarch, beeswax along with oil in a double boiler , and stir.

2. After melting completely, place the wax and oil mix in the food processor and allow to cool. (about 20 minutes)

3. When the oil mixture has become cool, but not completely soft, add the water, and then turn the food processor to low.

4. Once the lotion has become smooth, you can add essential oils.

5. After another few minutes, put the lotion into the pump dispenser.

6. Keep in the refrigerator and have fun!

This lotion is great for skin that is sensitive. Sweet almond oil as well as rose water and vital oils comprise the key ingredients in this recipe. Sweet almond oil can be beneficial for skin that is sensitive. It can be stored in the fridge for up 2 weeks.

The Fountain of Youth Lotion
Ingredients:

* 4 ounces of aloe Vera gel
* 4 8 ounces of neroli water
* 2 tablespoons of grapeseed oil
* 2 ounces avocado oil
* 2 1 ounces of beeswax
1. 1 tablespoon of Vitamin E oil

Five drops essential neroli oil

Method

1. A bowl is used to mix the aloe vera, neroli water as well as vitamin E oil.

2. Put oil and beeswax in the double boiler, stirring.

3. When the wax is completely melted, pour the wax and oil mix in the food processor and let it cool. (about 20 minutes)

4. When the oil mixture is cool, but not completely soft then switch the food processor to low, and slowly add the water.

5. When the lotion has become smooth, you can include the essential oils.

6. After another 15 minutes, transfer the lotion into the pump dispenser.

7. Place in a fridge and have fun!

This lotion is great for sensitive skin and anti-aging. Aloe vera and the oils and essential oil neroli are the most important and effective ingredients that make up this recipe. Grapeseed oil can be beneficial for skin that is aging. Keep it in the refrigerator for up to two weeks.

Tranquility Lotion

Ingredients:

* 4 cups of rose water
* 3 Oz of water containing neroli
* 2 ounces olive oil
* 2 pounds of beeswax

*1 teaspoon shea butter
• 1 teaspoon vitamin E oil
Five drops essential lavender oil
Three drops essential tea tree oil
Method
1. Within a container, mix the distilled water with Vitamin E oil.
2. Put oil and beeswax in the double boiler, stirring.
3. When the wax is completely melted, place the wax and oil mixture into the food processor , and allow it to cool.
4. When the oil mixture is cool, but not completely soft, switch the food processor off low, and slowly add the water.
5. When the lotion is smooth, you can add essential oils.
6. After another 15 minutes, transfer the lotion into the pump dispenser.
7. Keep in the refrigerator and have fun!
This lotion is suitable for skin that is sensitive. The rose water, the neroli water shea butter, and the essential oil blend are the active primary ingredients that make up this recipe. The recipe can be stored in the fridge for up 2 weeks.
Eczema Relief Lotion
Ingredients:
7oz water distilled

* 2 ounces coconut oil
* 2 ounces sweet almond oil
* 2 pounds of beeswax
* 1 teaspoon vitamin E oil
Five drops essential lavender oil
* Five drops essential tea tree oil
Method
1. Within a container, mix the distilled water with Vitamin E oil.
2. Put oil and beeswax in an oven double boiler. Stir.
3. After melting completely, place the wax and oil mixture into the food processor , and allow to cool. (about 20 minutes)
4. When the oil mixture has become cool, but not completely soft, switch the food processor to low, and slowly add the water.
5. Once the lotion has become smooth, you can add essential oils.
6. After another 15 minutes, transfer the lotion into the pump dispenser.
7. Place in a fridge and have fun!
This lotion is ideal for treating eczema and sensitive skin. The essential oils as well as the oil blend are the principal and active ingredients in this recipe. It can be effective in relieving eczema. It can be stored in the refrigerator for up to two weeks.
Cream Recipes

The Green Tea Refreshing Cream
Ingredients:
* 2 ounces coconut oil
Two teaspoons sweet almond oil
* 4 ounces of shea butter
* 1 teaspoon of beeswax
* Ten drops essential green tea oil
* Ten drops essential mint oil
Method
1. Combine all ingredients with the exception of oil essentials in a double-boiler and mix.
2. Once the melt is melted Add oil essentials.
3. Stir until creamy.
4. Pour into a glass jar.
5. Keep it in a dry place at room temperature. Enjoy!
The primary and active ingredients of this dish are the sweet almond oil as well as an essential blend of oils. Keep it in a dry location for up to six months.
Autumn Cream
Ingredients:
* 2 ounces olive oil
* 2 ounces coconut oil
* 2 1 ounces of shea butter
* 2 ounces of jojoba butter
* 1 one ounce of beeswax
* 5 drops of essential orange oil
Five drops essential fir needle oil

Five drops essential lemon oil

Method

1. Mix all the ingredients, excluding the essential oils into a double-boiler and mix.

2. Once the melt is melted Add all essential oils.

3. Stir until creamy.

4. Pour into a glass jar.

5. Keep it in a dry place at room temperature, and then enjoy!

The primary and active ingredients of this dish are butters, oils along with essential oils. Place them in a dry area for up to six months.

Sun Glow Cream

Ingredients:

* 4 tablespoons of coconut oil

* 4 8 ounces of mango butter

* 1 teaspoon of beeswax

* 10 drops of essential orange oil

Five drops essential grapefruit oil

Method

1. Combine all ingredients with the exception of the essential oils into a double-boiler and mix.

2. After melting Add oil essentials.

3. Stir until smooth.

4. Pour into a glass jar.

5. Keep it in a dry place at room temperature. Enjoy!

The primary and active ingredients of this recipe include mango butter, coconut oil as well as the essential oil mix. Place in a dry area for up to six months.

Forest Breeze Cream

Ingredients:

* 4 8 ounces of coconut oil
* 4 ounces of shea butter
* 1 one ounce of beeswax
* 10 drops essential jasmine oil

Five drops essential tea tree oil

Five drops essential eucalyptus oil

Method

1. Mix all ingredients with the exception of oil essentials in a double-boiler and mix.

2. Once the melt is melted then add all essential oils.

3. Stir until smooth.

4. Pour into a glass jar.

5. Place in a dry location at room temperature. Enjoy!

The primary and active ingredients in this recipe comprise Shea butter, coconut oil as well as the oil mix. Place in a dry area for up to six months.

Christmas Cream

Ingredients:

4. ounces Jojoba oil
* 4 tablespoons of shea butter
* 1 one ounce of beeswax

20 drops essential peppermint oil

Method

1. Mix all the ingredients, excluding oil essentials in a double-boiler and mix.
2. After melting Add all essential oils.
3. Stir until smooth.
4. Pour into a glass jar.
5. Keep it in a dry place at room temperature, and then enjoy!

The primary and active ingredients of this dish are Jojoba oil, shea butter as well as the essential peppermint oil. Place in a dry area for up to six months.

Chapter 6: Bath Bombs Recipes

Calendula bath bomb

The essential oil of calendula is abundant in carotene, fatty acids, Vitamin C, volatile and bitter compounds. It is a potent anti-inflammatory impact. Calendula oil is a great solution for skin irritation and acne.

Ingredients:

1. 1 tablespoon dry calendula

One teaspoon of essential oil of calendula

* 1/2 cup baking soda

1. 1 tablespoon olive oil

1. 1/2 Cup citric acid

* 3 tablespoons cornstarch

* 1 cup of salt

Method

Mix the dry calendula powder with the salt and cornstarch. Mix the ingredients carefully. Then , add essential calendula oil and olive oil. Mix the ingredients carefully. Use an electric hand mixer create the smooth mixture. Add baking soda, citric acid and then continue to stir the mixture using the aid by the hand mixer. Once you've got a great mixture , put it into the molds for bath bombs and press the mixture down. The bath bombs should be left for five days in an air-conditioned location. Remove the bath bombs from their molds and utilize them. Store the bath bombs in plastic bags and store them in an area that is dry and in your bathroom.

The pumpkin spicy bomb for bath

The pumpkin oil has huge amounts of polyunsaturated fatty acids, vitamins and essential for skin minerals. One of the most important

The main benefit of pumpkin oil is its ability to reduce the signs of aging. It is an oil well-known and is widely used in cosmetology industry.

The oil of the pumpkin has powerful rejuvenating, moisturizing, and rejuvenating effects.

Ingredients:
• 1 teaspoon pumpkin oil
* 1 teaspoon of cinnamon
* 1 teaspoon vanilla essential oil
*1 cup of cornstarch
*1 cup of citric acid
13 cup of sea salt
* 1/2 cup baking soda

Method

Mix the cornstarch with pumpkin oil. Make sure to stir the mixture thoroughly with the assistance of a hand whisker. Add the baking soda, cinnamon, as well as vanilla essential oil. The mixture should be stirred with a gentle stir. Then adding salt. Once you have an even and smooth wet mix, include citric acid. Utilize the spoon to stir the mixture until you have an even, smooth mass. Then , transfer the mixture to the molds designed for bath bombs or use muffin molds to complete this step. The mixture should be placed very securely in the molds. The molds should be left for at four hours at room that is warm. Remove the bath bombs out of the molds and put them in. The bath bombs should be kept in the wrapper in a dry location.

Bath bomb for Achy Muscles

An oil-based blend and arrowroot powders will aid in relaxing your stiff muscles. The Shi butter helps to make the skin soft and soft, and also nourishes it. These bath bombs are most suitable for bathing at night. Make sure to use it at least two times a week.

Ingredients:

* 1 teaspoon of arrowroot powder
* 1/2 cup baking soda
13 cup citric acid
Sea salt - 1/2 Cup
One teaspoon of almond oil
One teaspoon of Shi butter
1. 1 tablespoon cocoa oil
Method

Place the citric acid, baking soda and salt in a mixing bowl and stir the mixture gently. Then combine the almond oil, Shi butter and cocoa oil in a separate boil. Stir the mixture with the help of the hand mixer. After this, add arrowroot powder and continue to mix it for 30 seconds more. Then pour the liquid mixture in the dry mixture slowly. Stir it carefully will you get nice mixture. Then transfer the bath bomb mixture in the special bath bomb molds and press it tightly. Leave the bath bombs for 5 hours then remove them from the molds and wrap them in the wrapping paper. Keep the bath bombs in a dry place.

The Dead Sea mud bath bomb

Dead Sea mud can deal with skin ailments, nervous and cardiovascular systems, digestive, respiratory, renal, musculoskeletal system; mud helps to cope with women's and men's issues, as well as endocrine disorders.

Ingredients:

- 1 tablespoon the Dead Sea dry mud
- ½ cup the Dead Sea salt
- ½ cup baking soda
- ½ cup citric acid
- 1 tablespoon olive oil
- 1 teaspoon sweet almond oil

Method

Take the big mixing bowl and combine Dead Sea salt, mud, baking soda, and citric acid together in it. Stir the mixture. After this, pour the olive oil in the mixture and start to stir it carefully with the help of the spoon. Then add sweet almond oil and whisk the mixture. When you get little-wet mixture – transfer it in the special bath bomb's molds and press the mixture carefully in the molds. Leave the bath bombs for 7 hours. After this, remove the bath bombs from the molds and wrap them in plastic bags. Keep the bath bombs in a dry place.
Avocado oil bath bomb

Oil avocado contains a complex of fatty acids, which are directly involved in the development of human cells and normalize blood flow. The avocado oil is also necessary to adjust the fat metabolism and removes toxins, radionuclides, and heavy metals.

Ingredients:

- 1 teaspoon avocado oil
- ½ cup baking soda
- 1 teaspoon thyme oil
- 1 tablespoon cornstarch

- ½ cup citric acid
- ½ cup Epsom salt
- 1 teaspoon dry lemon zest

Method

Place the cornstarch, baking soda, citric acid, and Epsom salt together in a mixing bowl. Stir the mixture. Then add dry lemon zest and stir it again gently. Take a separate mixing bowl and pour thyme oil and avocado oil in it. Mix up the mass. After this, pour the liquid mixture into the dry mixture and whisk it constantly. Continue to whisk the mass till you get a smooth and nice mixture. Then take the muffin molds and place the bath bomb mixture in them. Press the mixture in the molds tightly. Then leave the muffin's molds for at least 6 hours. After this, remove the bath bombs from the molds and wrap them in the wrapping paper. Keep the bath bombs in a dry place in the bathroom.

Chapter 7: Removing Skin Tan

Remove skin tan with natural home remedies using either tomato or turmeric.
Removing Skin Tan:

• Tan refers to the skin darkening due to exposure to the UV radiation of the sun
• In many regions, tanning is often done intentionally by sun bathing or other artificial methods

Symptoms to look for:

• Darkening of the affected skin
• Presence of blisters in severe cases

Causes:

• Sun exposure facilitates production of vitamin D
• Excessive sun exposure can cause:
  o Sunburn
  o Skin cancer
  o Weak immune system
• Exposure to the sun damages melanin leading to brief skin darkening

Natural home remedy using tomatoes and lemon juice:

1. Crush 2 washed tomatoes into a puree
2. Add 4 tbsp lemon juice
3. Mix well
4. Apply on the tanned skin
5. Leave it for 20 min
6. Wash off with cold water
7. Do this for 15 days

Natural home remedy using lemon juice and turmeric powder:

1. Take 6 tbsp lemon juice
2. Add 2 tsp turmeric powder
3. Mix well to make paste
4. Apply on the tanned skin
5. Leave it for 30 min
6. Wash off with water

Tips:

• Rub potato slice on tanned skin for 5-10 min

Clear Skin Blemishes
Get clean & clear skin with natural home remedies by using either almonds or potatoes. Blemishes:

• A blemish is a discolored or a marked area on the skin

Causes:

• Marks may develop on skin due to skin conditions like boils, pimples or acne
• Other causes include,
  o Skin injuries
  o Age
  o Sun spots
  o Freckles
  o Moles

Natural home remedy using almonds and milk:

1. Soak 7-8 almonds in water for 12 hours
2. Peel and crush them
3. Add a little milk to make a paste
4. Apply on blemishes
5. Leave it overnight
6. Wash with cold water in the morning
7. Do this for at least 2 weeks

Natural home remedy using potato:

1. Take a potato slice
2. Rub on the affected area for 10 min

3. Do this 2-3 times a day

Natural home remedy using mint leaves:

1. Crush some mint leaves into a fine paste
2. Apply this paste on the blemishes
3. Leave it for 20 min
4. Wash off with cold water

Acne
Treat acne with natural home remedies by using either garlic or coriander leaves.
Acne:

• Acne affects 60% of youngsters between 12 to 24 years of age
• It causes embarrassment, depression and lack of confidence

Symptoms to look for:

• Whiteheads
• Blackheads
• Pimples
• Red and itchy rashes

Causes:

• The body is unable to remove toxins through excretion leading to contamination of the bloodstream. This can be due to:
  o Constipation
  o Irregular bowel movement
  o Irregular meal timings
  o Excess starch, sugar, oil and fat consumption

Natural home remedy using garlic:

1. Garlic contains allicin, which is a natural antibiotic
2. Take 2-3 garlic cloves
3. Crush them to make a paste
4. Apply this paste on the affected parts of the skin
5. For sensitive skin, mix yogurt in the garlic paste before applying

Natural home remedy using garlic:

1. Consume three cloves of garlic everyday for 1 month

Natural home remedy using coriander leaves and turmeric powder:

1. Take a handful of washed coriander leaves

2. Crush them finely

3. Place the paste on a sieve and press to extract the juice

4. Add a pinch of turmeric powder

5. Mix well

6. Apply this mixture on the face every night

Skin Pigmentation

Treat skin pigmentation with natural home remedies using yogurt, turmeric or oatmeal.

Skin Pigmentation:

• Skin pigmentation is a condition wherein dark patches appear on the skin

• Although not life threatening, it can be a detriment to self-esteem

Symptoms to look for:

• Discoloration of the skin

• Presence of patches

Causes:

• Melanin provides color to skin

• Excessive production of melanin causes dark patches

Natural home remedy using tomato, oatmeal and yogurt:

1. Crush 1 tomato
2. Press on a sieve and extract its juice
3. Add 2 tsp oatmeal to it
4. Add ½ tsp yogurt
5. Apply on the patches
6. Allow it to dry naturally
7. Leave it for 15-20 min
8. Wash off with lukewarm water
9. Do this every day

Natural home remedy using turmeric powder and lemon juice:

1. Take 1 tsp turmeric powder
2. Add 1 tsp lemon juice
3. Mix well
4. Apply on the affected area
5. Leave it for 15 min to dry
6. Wash off with cold water
7. Do not expose skin to the sun immediately after this
8. Application at bedtime is advisable

Regular Skin Care
Regular Skin Care with natural home remedies by using either banana or yogurt.
Care for Normal Facial Skin (Face Masks for Cleansing and Fairness):

• The skin type is considered normal, when there is a right oil and moisture balance
• In normal skin,
  o Skin tone is even
  o There are usually no spots or blemishes
• Use natural face masks to get a glowing and a healthy skin

Natural face masks using banana, yogurt and honey:

1. Mash half a banana
2. Add 2 tbsp of yogurt
3. Add 1 tbsp of honey
4. Mix well
5. Apply on the face taking care to avoid the eyes
6. Leave for 15 min
7. Wash off with cold water

Natural face masks using yogurt and orange:

1. Take 1 tbsp of yogurt
2. Add juice of ¼ of an orange
3. Mix well
4. Apply on the face taking care to avoid the eyes
5. Leave for 5 min and then wash it off

Acne Scars

Get rid of acne scars with natural home remedies using Aloe vera leaves or honey, lemon juice and almond oil.

Acne Scars:

• Popping or scratching acne can leave scars

Natural home remedy using aloe vera:

1. Take an aloe vera leaf
2. Peel the outer green covering
3. Extract the gel from inside
4. Apply the gel 2 times a day
5. Leave it for 30 minutes
6. Wash it off

Natural home remedy using honey, lemon juice, almond oil and milk:

1. Take 1 tbsp of honey
2. Add 1 tbsp lemon juice
3. Add 1 tbsp almond oil
4. Add 2 tbsp of milk
5. Mix Well
6. Apply on the affected area

Allergies

Treat allergies with natural home remedies using honey or juice of carrot, cucumber and beetroot.

Allergies:

• Allergies occur when the immune system reacts abnormally to certain stimuli
• These stimuli are referred to as allergens

Symptoms to look for:

Reaction to allergens vary in individuals and can cause,

• Hives
• Rashes
• Anaphylactic attack in severe cases

There are 3 types of allergies

1. Respiratory allergies which lead to:

• Sneezing
• Coughing
• Watering of eyes and nose
• Asthma

2. Food allergies which lead to

- Diarrhoea
- Flatulence
- Eczema
- Skin rashes
- Swelling of throat

3. Contact allergies which cause:

- Itching inflammation
- Burning sensation
- Blisters

Causes:

- The Immune system incorrectly perceives some substances as a threat
- Respiratory allergies are caused by airborne allergens like dust, pollen, etc
- Food allergy is are caused as an adverse reaction to certain food items
- Contact allergy is caused by skin's reaction to some metals, fragrances or latex

Natural home remedy using carrot juice, beetroot juice and cucumber juice:

1. Take 250 ml carrot juice

2. Add 100 ml beetroot juice
3. Add 100 ml cucumber juice
4. Mix well
5. Have once everyday
6. This helps reduce allergic reaction and soothes existing allergies

Natural home remedy using lemon and honey:

Lemon helps flush toxins from the body. It is an antibiotic and has anti-allergic properties

1. Take 1 glass lukewarm water
2. Squeeze ½ lemon in it
3. Add 1 tsp honey
4. Mix well
5. Drink on an empty stomach

Oily Skin Care
Treat oily skin with natural home remedies by using either apples or milk.
Care for Oily Skin:

• Oily skin is a result of overactive oil producing glands in the skin
• This makes the skin thick and greasy

Symptoms to look for:

- Blackheads
- Whiteheads
- Pimples
- Skin spots

Natural home remedy using apple and honey:

1. De-seed and crush 1 apple
2. Add 4 tbsp honey
3. Mix well
4. Apply on the face
5. Wash it off after 10 min

Natural home remedy using ice and milk:

1. Dip 1 cube of ice in milk
2. Rub the ice on the face
3. Keep dipping the ice in the milk and rubbing on your face for 5-10 min

Blackheads
Treat blackheads with natural home remedies by using either coriander leaves or groundnut oil.
Blackheads:

- Blackheads are one of the most common forms of acne

Symptoms to look for:

• Dark spots appearing around:
  o Forehead
  o Nose
  o Chin area

Causes:

• Oil producing glands in the skin produce excess oil
• This leads to expansion and thickening of skin pores
• Oil accumulates in the pores and hardens
• Air reacts with this oil, turning it black in color

Natural home remedy using lemon juice and cinnamon powder:

1. Take 1 tsp lemon juice
2. Add 1 tsp cinnamon powder
3. Mix well
4. Apply on the affected area
5. Leave it for 15-20 min
6. Repeat 2-3 times a day

Natural home remedy using coriander leaves and turmeric powder:

1. Crush a handful of washed coriander leaves
2. Press it on a sieve
3. Extract 1 tsp juice
4. Add 1 tsp turmeric powder to make paste
5. Apply this paste on the face every night
6. Leave it for 30 min
7. Wash off with lukewarm water

Tips:

• Avoid oil-based skin products

Moles
Treat moles with natural home remedies by using either coriander leaves or pineapple.
Moles:

• Moles are round in shape, plain or raised spots on the skin
• They are harmless but their appearance can be a cosmetic concern
• Moles are present during birth but grow and darken with time

Symptoms to look for:

• Usually moles are black or brown in color
• Some can even be red or pink

• Moles could also have hair growing out of them

Causes:

• Melanin gives the skin its color
• Over-active melanocytes in the body produce excess melanin resulting in moles

Natural home remedy using coriander leaves:

1. Crush some coriander leaves to make paste
2. Apply this paste on the spots
3. Let it stay overnight

Natural home remedy using pineapple:

1. Cut a pineapple
2. Rub on the moles for about 5-10 min
3. Do this several times a day

Natural home remedy using garlic:

1. Crush a few garlic cloves to make paste
2. Apply this paste on the mole
3. Hold it for 30 min using a bandage or cloth
4. Do this every day for 2-3 weeks

Natural home remedy using cashew nuts:

1. Take ½ bowl of crushed cashew nuts
2. Add some water to make a paste
3. Apply this paste on moles
4. Applying this paste regularly will help fade the marks

Stretch Marks

Remove stretch marks with natural home remedies by using apricots, aloe vera or lavender oil.

Stretch Marks:

- Stretch marks usually appear on:
  o Abdomen
  o Back
  o Waist
  o Arms
  o Hips
  o Breast
  o Lower back
  o Legs

Symptoms to look for:

- Stretch marks are thick red or purple lines on the skin
- Over time, these lines fade to white or silver in color

Causes:

• Skin is made up of elastin, which is a soft elastic tissue. It makes the skin soft, supple and stretchable.
 Over-stretching of skin damages elastin resulting in stretch marks.
• Sudden weight change
• Rapid body growth during teenage
• Pregnancy

Natural home remedy using apricots:

1. Cut and remove seeds of 2-3 apricots
2. Crush them to paste
3. Apply this paste on the marks
4. Leave it for 20 min
5. Wash it off with lukewarm water
6. Repeat this regularly for 1 month

Natural home remedy using aloe vera:

1. Aloe vera has plant collagen which repairs the skin.
2. Remove the thorns and outer skin of a few aloe vera leaves
3. Extract the gel from inside
4. Apply this gel on the stretch marks

5. Leave it for 2 hr
6. Wash it off with normal water

Natural home remedy using lavender oil, chamomile oil and almond oil:

1. Take ½ tsp lavender oil
2. Add ½ tsp chamomile oil
3. Add 2 tsp almond oil
4. Mix well
5. Apply on the stretch marks

Tips:

• Apply petroleum jelly on the abdomen during pregnancy
  o But do not do this without consulting your doctor

Dry Skin Care
Treat dry skin care with natural home remedies by using either wheat flour or honey.
Care for Dry Facial Skin (Face Masks for Cleansing and Fairness):

• A good skin is a symbol of good health
• Skin requires as much care as any other part of our body

• Use natural face masks to get glowing and healthy facial skin

Symptoms to look for:

• Dry Skin,
• Wrinkles easily
• Appears parched
• Ages rapidly
• Flakes often

Causes:

• Lack of oil and moisture in the skin

Natural face mask using wheat flour, turmeric powder and mustard oil:

1. Take 4 tbsp of wheat flour
2. Add ½ tsp of turmeric powder
3. Add 1 tsp of mustard oil
4. Add water to make a paste
5. Apply the paste on the face taking care to avoid the eyes
6. Leave it to dry for 10 min
7. Remove the dried mask by scrubbing it with your palms
8. After 30 min, wash off with lukewarm water

Natural face mask using honey and milk:

1. Take 2 tbsp of honey
2. Add 2 tsp of milk
3. Mix well
4. Apply on the face and neck taking care to avoid the eyes
5. Leave it for 20 min
6. Wash off with lukewarm water

Wrinkles
Prevent and treat wrinkles with natural home remedies using egg white.
Wrinkles:

• Skin loses its elasticity with age
• Wrinkles are creases caused in skin when it thins and sags due to old age
• Wrinkles first appear near the eye and with age, they appear on cheeks, lips, neck and hand

Causes:

• Rough environmental conditions can cause premature wrinkles
• Chemicals present in the smoke can destroy skin cells

Natural home remedy using egg whites:

1. Egg whites contain vitamins, which help tighten skin
2. Apply egg whites on wrinkle prone areas
3. Leave for 20 min
4. Wash with lukewarm water

Natural home remedy using avocado, fresh cream, flaxseeds and honey:

1. Crush and make paste of ½ an avocado
2. Add 2 tbsp of fresh cream
3. Add 2 tsp of flaxseeds
4. Add 1 tbsp of honey
5. Mix well
6. Apply on the skin and leave it for 1 hr
7. Wash with cold water
8. This mixture is a natural moisturizer

Natural home remedy using papaya and banana:

This remedy is especially for men

1. Blend papaya and banana together
2. Apply on the skin
3. Leave it for 20 min
4. Wash it off with lukewarm water

Papaya has chemicals, which remove dead skin cells. Banana provides necessary nutrients for healthy skin

Tips:

- Have a balanced diet consisting of:
  o Fruits
  o Vegetables
  o Whole grain foods
  o Seeds
  o Nuts
  o Legumes
- Drink 8-10 glasses of water every day to keep skin hydrated
- Avoid:
  o Alcohol
  o Caffeine
  o Smoking
- Use a sunscreen before stepping out in the sun

Dry Skin
Treat dry skin with natural home remedies by using either bananas or barley flour.
Dry Skin:

- Dry skin occurs due to loss of skin moisture
- This usually occurs during cold weather

- For some, dry skin is a chronic problem
- If ignored, fissures or deep cracks can develop on the skin which may cause bleeding

Symptoms to look for:

- Dry flaking skin
- Lines and wrinkles on the skin
- Itchiness
- White lines on scratching

Causes:

- Bathing in hot water multiple times a day
- Swimming
- Overexposure to sunlight
- Psoriasis, a medical condition of the skin
- Sitting for long in artificially heated or cooled rooms where humidity levels   are low

Natural home remedy using bananas and honey:

1. Take 2 mashed bananas
2. Add 2 tbsp of honey
3. Mix well
4. Apply on dry skin
5. Leave it for 20 min
6. Wash off with warm water

Natural home remedy using barley flour, turmeric powder and mustard oil:

1. Take 2 tbsp of barley flour
2. Add 1 tsp of turmeric powder
3. Add 2 tsp of mustard oil
4. Add water
5. Mix well to make a paste
6. Apply this paste on the affected parts of the skin
7. Leave it for 10 min
8. Scrub it off with your palms
9. Bathe with lukewarm water

This will make the skin soft, fair and silky

Natural home remedy using egg yolk:

1. Take 1 egg yolk
2. Beat it lightly
3. Apply this on the dry skin
4. Leave it for 20 min before washing

Tips:

• Massage using olive oil or almond oil
• Drink 8 to 10 glasses of water every day as these flushes out the toxins

• Use a moisturizer regularly

Cracked Heel
Treat cracked heel with natural home remedies by using either lemons or bananas.
Cracked Heel:

• Cracked heel is the result of neglect and lack of moisturizing of the heels
• The heels develop deep cuts which may become painful

Symptoms to look for:

• Red or flaky patches on the heels are the first signs
• Cracks on skin which may bleed

Causes:

• Feet expand sideways due to excessive pressure. Cracks may develop due to:
  o Dry skin
  o Zinc and omega-3 fatty acid deficiency

Natural home remedy using bananas:

1. Crush ripe bananas to make paste
2. Apply this paste on the cracks

3. Leave it for 10 min
4. Wash off with water
5. Do this every day

Natural home remedy using margosa leaves and turmeric powder:

1. Crush a handful of margosa leaves to make paste
2. Add 3 tsp turmeric powder
3. Mix well
4. Apply the paste on cracks
5. Leave it for 30 min
6. Wash off with water
7. Dry with a soft cloth
8. Do this twice everyday

Natural home remedy using lemon:

1. Cut a lemon into half
2. Rub the lemon on your feet
3. Squeeze the lemon and apply the juice while rubbing
4. Continue rubbing for 5 min
5. Lightly scrub feet with a loofah or soft brush
6. Wash feet with water
7. Lemon juice is mildly acidic and helps remove dead skin cells.

Tips:

• Avoid wearing sandals with open backs as these facilitate sideways
 expansion of feet causing cracks
• Do not stand barefoot in damp areas for long time as this can make the skin dry

Itching
Get relief from itching with natural home remedies by using either cinnamon or coconut oil.
Itching:

• Itching refers to the urge to scratch
• Itching is a form of skin irritation
• Regular itching can lead to bruises and make the skin sore
• Itching can affect a local area on skin or can be present throughout the body

Symptoms to look for:

• Constant urges to scratch
• Itching can lead to
 o Bruises
 o Sore skin

Causes:

- Skin ailments like:
  - o Skin rashes
  - o Skin lesions
  - o Blisters
  - o Dry skin
  - o Eczema
- Pregnancy
- Menopause
- Contact with harsh detergents and solvents
- Allergens
- Insect bites or stings
- Lack of hygiene

Natural home remedy using cinnamon and honey:

1. Take 2 tsp cinnamon powder
2. Add 2 tsp honey
3. Mix well
4. Apply on the affected area
5. Leave it for 10-15 min
6. Wash off with water
7. Do this 3 times a day

Natural home remedy using coconut oil and lemon juice:

1. Take 6 tbsp coconut oil

2. Add 4 tbsp lemon juice
3. Mix well
4. Heat the mixture till it turns lukewarm
5. Apply on the affected area
6. Leave it overnight

Natural home remedy using corn starch:

1. Take 3 tbsp corn starch
2. Add some water to make a paste
3. Mix well
4. Apply on the affected area
5. Leave it for 15 min
6. Wash off with water
7. Repeat this 3 times a day

Leucoderma
Treat leucoderma with natural home remedies by using either turmeric powder or walnuts.
Leucoderma:

• Leucoderma is a skin disease wherein white patches appear on the skin

Symptoms to look for:

• White spots on skin, which grow in size over time
• Continuous loss of skin pigment

Causes:

- Gastric disorders
- Excessive stress
- Burn injuries
- Perspiration disorders

Natural home remedy using turmeric powder and mustard oil:

1. Take 1 tsp of turmeric powder
2. Add 2 tsp of mustard oil
3. Mix well
4. Apply paste on affected areas
5. Leave for 15-20 min
6. Apply 3-4 times everyday

Natural home remedy using walnuts:

1. Crush some walnuts into powder
2. Take 2 tsp of this walnut powder
3. Add little water
4. Mix well
5. Apply this paste on affected area 3-4 times a day
6. Leave it for 15-20 min
7. Wash it off

Natural home remedy using margosa leaves and honey:

1. Crush a handful of washed margosa leaves
2. Put the paste on a sieve
3. Press the paste to extract the juice
4. Take 2 tsp of this juice
5. Add 1 tsp honey
6. Mix well
7. Drink 3 times everyday

Chicken Pox
Treat chicken pox with natural home remedies by using either green peas or carrots.
Chicken Pox:

• Chicken pox is a viral infection
• The most prominent symptom is the appearance of red spots and rashes on skin
• It is a highly contagious condition

Symptoms to look for:

• Rashes or tiny red spots on the skin
  o These appear mostly on the upper back or chest
  o As infection grows rashes spread to face and lower extremities
• Overtime,

o Rashes get filled with fluid

o Thick crust develops

• As some of these rashes dry, new ones come up
• Itchy blisters
• Mild fever
• Headache
• Weakness

Causes:

• The condition may spread if one comes in contact with,

o Cough or sneeze of an infected person

o Fluid from the chickenpox blister
• Lack of vaccination for chickenpox

Natural home remedy using green peas:

1. Take 200 g green peas
2. Boil them in water
3. Drain the water
4. Crush the peas to make a paste
5. Apply this paste on the affected area
6. Leave it for 1 hr

Natural home remedies using baking soda:

1. Baking soda helps control the itching

2. Take 1 bowl of water
3. Add 3 tbsp baking soda
4. Mix well
5. Use a sponge to apply on the skin
6. Make sure that the soda dries on skin

Natural home remedies using carrots and coriander leaves:

1. Take 100 g chopped carrots
2. Add 60 g fresh coriander leaves
3. Add them in 500 ml water and boil till water reduces to half
4. Drink this soup once a day
5. Add salt and pepper for taste

Tips:

• Vaccinate your child for chicken pox
• Avoid itching or scratching the blisters as it can aggravate the condition. It can also leave permanent scars on the skin

Eczema
Treat eczema with natural home remedies by using either margosa leaves (neem) or mustard oil.
Eczema (Dermatitis):

- Eczema is the inflammation of the skin
- It is common amongst children
- It is also known as dermatitis

Symptoms to look for:

- Severe itching
- Dryness
- Redness
- Skin flaking
- Small bumps on the forehead, neck and cheeks

Causes:

- Hereditary factors, specifically in families where there is a history of ailments like:
  - o Asthma
  - o Hay fever
- Irregular blood circulation in the legs
- Vitamin B6 deficiency
- This condition is aggravated by harsh chemicals like:
  - o Detergents
  - o Solvents
  - o Smoke
  - o Chemicals
- Other irritants
  - o Changes in weather

o Extreme stress
o Heat

Natural home remedy using margosa leaves and turmeric powder:

1. Crush some margosa leaves
2. Take 1 tbsp of this pulp
3. Add 1 tsp of turmeric powder
4. Mix well to make a paste
5. Apply on the affected areas

Natural home remedy using mustard oil and margosa leaves:

1. Take 200 g of mustard oil
2. Add 50 g of margosa leaves
3. Heat the mustard oil
4. Stop when the leaves turn black
5. Allow the oil to cool
6. Strain the oil and apply on the affected area 3 times a day

Natural home remedy using aloe vera:

1. Remove the outer skin of aloe vera leaves
2. Extract gel from inside
3. Apply this gel on the affected skin
4. Leave it for 30 min

5. Do this 2 times a day

Tips:

• Wash clothes thoroughly to remove any residual detergent or other solvents

Boils
Treat boils with natural home remedies by using either cumin seeds or onions.
Boils:

• Boils occur when there's an infection in the hair follicle or an oil gland on the skin
• This infection leads to red pus filled boils on the skin
• The areas usually affected are:
  o Face
  o Neck
  o Buttocks
  o Armpits
  o Thighs

Symptoms to look for:

• Boils are,
  o Itchy
  o Painful
  o Irritating

Causes:

• Bacterial infection of the skin
• Consumption of antibiotics over a prolonged period of time
• Medical conditions which can lead to boils:
  o Diabetes
  o Blood disorders
  o Obesity
  o Anaemia

Natural home remedy using cumin seeds:

1. Take 50 g cumin seeds
2. Add a little water
3. Crush to make a paste
4. Apply on the boils

Natural home remedy using onion and garlic:

1. Take 1 chopped onion
2. Add 2-3 chopped garlic cloves
3. Press this on a sieve
4. Extract juice
5. Apply this on boils 4-5 times everyday

Natural home remedy using milk cream, vinegar and turmeric powder:

1. Take 1 tsp of milk cream
2. Add 1 tsp of vinegar
3. Add 1 tsp of turmeric powder
4. Mix well
5. Apply this paste on the boils

Tips:

• Unhygienic conditions facilitate bacterial activities and can lead to boils
• Choose soap which suits your skin
• Bathe regularly
• Always apply a moisturizer after bathing

Chapter 8: Sunburn

Treat sunburn with natural home remedies using papaya, cucumber or tomatoes.
Sunburn:

• One may suffer from sunburn while pursuing outdoor activities like running, hiking or swimming

Symptoms to look for:

• Red rashes
• Tenderness
• Blisters
• Peeling skin
• Extreme sunburn can also result in:
  o Fever
  o Chills
  o Nausea
  o Vomiting
  o Flu

Causes:

• Sunburn is caused by the action of ultra-violet rays of the sun on the skin

Natural home remedy using oatmeal, papaya and honey:

1. Take 1 cup chopped papaya
2. Crush the papaya to a paste
3. Add 2 tbsp oatmeal
4. Add 1 tbsp honey
5. Mix well
6. Apply this on your skin
7. Leave it for 30 min
8. Wash off with cold water

Natural home remedy using lemons and honey:

1. Squeeze juice of 2 lemons
2. Add to it 3 tbsp honey
3. Mix well
4. Apply this mixture on the skin
5. Leave for 20 min
6. Wash off with water
7. Do this 2 times a day

Natural home remedy using cucumber and lemon juice:

1. Cut 1 cucumber into small pieces
2. Crush it to make a paste
3. Press this paste on a sieve
4. Extract its juice

5. Add 2 tbsp lemon juice
6. Mix well
7. Apply on the affected area with cotton
8. Wash off after 15 min

Natural home remedy using tomatoes and yogurt:

1. Crush 2-3 tomatoes
2. Press the pulp on a sieve
3. Extract the juice
4. Add 1 tbsp yogurt
5. Mix well
6. Apply on the affected area
7. Leave for 15-20 min
8. Do this 2 times a day

Freckles
Treat freckles with natural home remedies by using either lemons or bananas.
Freckles:

• Freckles are dark spots on the skin
• They occur mostly on the face, around the nose
• Medically harmless, freckles are common amongst fair skinned people

Causes:

- Hereditary factors
- Constant exposure to sunlight

Natural home remedy using banana and mint leaves:

1. Mash 1 ripe banana
2. Add 2 tsp of crushed mint leaves
3. Apply this paste on the freckles
4. When pack begins to melt, wash it off

Natural home remedy using lemon juice, salt and honey:

1. Take 1 tbsp lemon juice
2. Add a pinch of salt
3. Add 1 tbsp honey
4. Apply the mixture on the freckles
5. Leave it for 10 min
6. Make sure that this doesn't enter the eyes
7. Wash off with normal water

Natural home remedy using potato and buttermilk:

1. Soak potato slices in buttermilk
2. Rub the slices on the freckles for 5 min
3. Repeat 3 times a week

Psoriasis

• Psoriasis mostly occurs between 15-30 years of age

Symptoms to look for:

• Red scaly patches, which usually appear around:
  o Torso
  o Knees
  o Elbows
• Dry skin
• Itching
• Silver flaky scales
• Joint pain
• Genital lesions in men
• Discoloration of nails
• Excessive dandruff

Causes:

• Skin cells grow, die and fall off in a period of 1 month
• In psoriasis, the cycle is reduced to 4 days
• Skin cells do not develop properly nor fall off easily
• This leads to dry, scaly patches

Natural home remedy using cabbage:

1. Take 1 bowl of crushed cabbage leaves
2. Take a bowl of hot water
3. Place the bowl of cabbage leaves inside the bowl of hot water, till the
   leaves turn lukewarm
4. Apply the lukewarm cabbage leaves on the affected area
5. Cover with a soft woollen cloth
6. Wrap with an elastic bandage for 2-3 hr

Natural home remedy using bitter gourd and lemons:

1. Take 1 glass of bitter gourd juice
2. Add 1 tsp lemon juice
3. Mix well
4. Drink this every day on an empty stomach
5. Have this for 4-6 months

Tips:

• Baking soda reduces itching
  o Add 2 tbsp baking soda to 1 bowl water
  o Soak a towel in this mixture, wring it out and apply on the skin as a
     compress

• Expose your skin to the morning sun as its effective in reducing skin inflammation and scaling

Ringworm
Treat ringworm infection with natural home remedies using either papaya seeds or basil leaves.
Ringworm:

• Ringworm is a common skin disease
• It's caused by fungal growth on the skin
• Ringworm is a contagious condition

Symptoms to look for:

• Round or oval patches
• Itching

Causes:

• Scratching spreads infection to other parts of the body
• It spreads through contact of utilising articles of infected people
• Risk of ringworm increases in:
  o Warm and humid condition
  o If one has a weak immune system

Natural home remedy using papaya:

1. Raw papaya is an effective remedy for ringworm
2. Separate the seeds from the papaya
3. Dry the seeds in the sun for 4-5 hr
4. Crush the dried seeds
5. Add little water to make a paste
6. Apply on the infected area
7. Do this 2-3 times a day

• Rubbing papaya on the infection is also useful. Rub it for 10-15 min, 3 times a day

Natural home remedy using mustard seeds:

1. Take 1 tsp of crushed mustard seeds
2. Add little water to make a paste
3. Apply on affected area
4. Wash after 60 min with lukewarm water

Natural home remedy using basil leaves:

1. Crush some basil leaves
2. Press the paste on a sieve and extract its juice
3. Take 2 tsp of this juice
4. Apply on the infected area using cotton

Jock Itch

Treat jock itch with natural home remedies by using either garlic or honey.

Jock Itch:

• Jock itch is a fungal infection which develops in the groin area
• The infection extends to the inner thighs and buttocks

Symptoms to look for:

• Red rashes on skin
• Rashes are scaly and raised
• Older rashes turn reddish brown
• Development of pus

Causes:

• The infection occurs in warm and moist conditions
• It's common in people who:
  o Are overweight
  o Sweat excessively

Natural home remedy using garlic and honey:

1. Crush 6-7 garlic cloves

2. Add 1 tsp honey
3. Mix well
4. Apply on the infected area
5. Allow the paste to dry
6. Wash off with normal water

Natural home remedy using baking soda paste:

1. Take 2 tsp baking soda
2. Add a little water to make a paste
3. Apply on the infected area
4. Leave it for 20 min
5. Wash off with water

Natural home remedy using salt:

1. Fill a bathtub with water
2. Mix 250 g of salt in it
3. Soak yourself in water for 15 min
4. Repeat 2 times every day
5. Salt dries up the blisters.

Natural home remedy using coconut oil:

1. Apply coconut oil on the infected area
2. Do this twice a day

Peeling Skin

Treat peeling skin with natural home remedies using either mint leaves or cucumber.
Peeling Skin:

• The outer layer of the skin suffers wear and tear due to:
  o Friction
  o Exposure to sun
  o Humidity
• Every month the old skin is replaced by a new one
  o During this time, peeling skin is normal

Symptoms to look for:

• Peeling skin becomes a problem when the condition becomes chronic and affects one frequently

Causes:

• Eczema
• Sun burns
• Psoriasis
• Dry skin

Natural home remedy using cucumber:

1. Peel and crush 1 cucumber to paste

2. Apply the paste on the affected area
3. Leave it for 15 min
4. Wash off with warm water
5. Do this regularly

Natural home remedy using mint leaves:

1. Crush a few washed mint leaves
2. Press on a sieve and extract their juice
3. Apply this juice on the peeled skin to keep it hydrated

This is highly effective for eczema and dermatitis patients.

Natural home remedy using turmeric, sandalwood, honey and olive oil:

1. Take 1 tsp turmeric powder
2. Add 1 tsp sandalwood powder
3. Add 1 tsp honey
4. Add olive oil to make a paste
5. Mix well
6. Apply on the affected area
7. Wash and dry after 30 min

Tips:

• Drink 8-10 glasses of water every day

• Wear a sunscreen before stepping out in sun
• Use mild soap for bathing

Corns

Treat corns with natural home remedies using either licorice or papaya.

Corn:

• Corn is a raised bump or a rough patch on the skin
• The tiny toe is most susceptible to corn
• Corn may develop on other fingers as well

Symptoms to look for:

• Raised bump or a rough patch on the skin

Causes:

• Increased pressure and friction on the feet causes the skin around the affected area to harden up and for a
  corn. It could be due to:
    o Tight footwear
    o Hard shoe soles
    o High heels
    o Walking or standing for a long time

Natural home remedy using liquorice and mustard oil:

1. Take 2 tbsp liquorice powder
2. Add 2 tsp mustard oil
3. Mix well
4. Apply on corns before sleeping
5. Let it stay overnight
6. Apply this for a month

Natural home remedy using papaya:

1. Crush papaya to make paste
2. Apply this paste on the corn
3. Wrap it with a cloth
4. Leave it overnight
5. Do this for a month

Tips:

• Apply castor oil 3-4 times a day
• Wear comfortable footwear. It shouldn't be tight around toes or have a hard base
• Buy shoes with extra padding

Rosacea
Treat rosacea with natural home remedies using fenugreek seeds or licorice powder.
Rosacea:

• Rosacea is a chronic skin condition usually affecting the face
• This condition is often mistaken for acne or eczema
• People with lighter skin tones are more prone to this disease

Symptoms to look for:

• Red patches
• Swelling of face
• Brief burning sensation on skin multiple times during the day
• Irritation in the eye
• Watery eyes
• Thick and dry skin
• Swollen eyelids

Causes:

• Swelling of the blood vessels beneath the skin
• Factors which aggravate rosacea are:
  o Sunlight
  o Spicy food
  o Alcohol
  o Stress
  o Sinus infection
  o Extreme temperatures

Natural home remedy using fenugreek seeds, ginger and honey:

1. Take 2 tbsp fenugreek seeds
2. Add 1 L water
3. Allow the mixture to simmer for 30 min
4. Strain the liquid
5. Take 2 tsp ginger paste
6. Press the paste on a sieve and extract juice
7. Add the ginger juice to the strained liquid
8. Add 1 tsp honey
9. Mix well
10. Sip 1 glass of this mixture every morning
11. Do this for 15 days to prevent reoccurrence of rosacea

Natural home remedy using licorice powder, honey and aloe vera:

1. Take 1 tsp licorice powder
2. Add 1 tsp honey
3. Remove thorns and outer skin of an aloe vera leaf
4. Extract gel from inside
5. Add 1 tsp of this gel to the mixture
6. Mix well
7. Apply on the face
8. Leave it for 15 min
9. Wash off with lukewarm water

Tips:

• Avoid skin products with mineral oils, alcohol and fragrance
• Avoid spicy and sugar based foods

Athlete's Foot
Treat athlete's foot with natural home remedies using garlic or cornstarch.
Athlete's Foot:

• Athlete's foot is a condition caused by a group of fungi called dermatophytes

Symptoms to look for:

• Itching between the toes
• Scaly, reddish and rough skin
• Moist, white lesions leading to pain and discomfort
• Pungent smell
• Infection may spread to nails making them thick and yellow in color

Causes:

• Wearing closed footwear for long periods of time leads to collection of sweat

• The moist conditions facilitate fungal growth

Natural home remedy using baking soda:

1. Take 2 tbsp of baking soda
2. Add some water to make a paste
3. Apply the paste on the infected area
4. Once dry, wash it off
5. Dry your feet thoroughly with a towel

Natural home remedy using corn starch:

1. Take some corn starch
2. Apply on the affected area with cotton
3. Wash after 15 minutes

Natural home remedy using garlic:

1. Crush 5-7 garlic cloves to make a paste
2. Massage on the infected area
3. Leave it for 10 minutes
4. Wash with normal water

Natural home remedy using vinegar:

1. Vinegar is acidic and kills fungus
2. Take 1 part vinegar and 4 parts water
3. Mix in a tub
4. Soak your feet in it for 20-30 min

5. Do this twice everyday

Tips:

• Dry your feet after bathing
• Clean your shoes regularly
• Wear open-toed sandals if you sweat a lot

Burns
Treat burns with natural home remedies by using either aloe vera gel or turmeric.
Burns:

• A burn is caused by accidently coming in contact with:
   o Fire
   o Hot fluids
   o Chemicals
• It's one of the most common forms of injuries

Symptoms to look for:

• Burns are divided into 3 categories:
• First degree burns:
   o Minor skin inflammation
   o Redness of skin
   o Swelling
   o Tender skin
• Second degree burns:

o They go deeper in the skin
o Blisters
o Pain and inflammation
• Third degree burns:
o They are the most severe
o They destroy the affected skin area

Natural home remedy using aloe vera:

1. De-thorn and remove the outer skin of an aloe vera leaf
2. Extract aloe vera gel from inside
3. Apply aloe vera gel on the affected area
4. Leave it for 30 min
5. Repeat twice a day

Natural home remedy using egg white:

1. Take 1 egg white
2. Apply it on the affected area
3. Wash after 10 min

Natural home remedy using turmeric powder and mustard oil:

1. Take 1 tsp turmeric powder
2. Add 1 tbsp mustard oil
3. Mix well
4. Apply on the burn

5. Leave it for 30 min
6. Do this twice a day

Tips:

• Immediately reduce the temperature of the skin by putting chilled water on it. Do not apply ice directly
  on the skin
• Only first degree burns should be treated at home
• If rose water is easily available, wash the affected area with it

Cold Sores
Treat cold sores with natural home remedies using tea or baking soda.
Cold Sores (Fever Blisters):

• Cold sores are small and painful fluid-filled blisters
• They appear on:
  o Lips
  o Gums
  o Tongue
  o Throat
  o Chin
• Cold sores are also referred to as fever blisters

Symptoms to look for:

- Reddish gums
- Swollen gums
- Bleeding
- Difficulty in swallowing

Causes:

- Entry of the herpes simplex virus
- The immune system cannot eliminate the herpes virus and hence the condition can keep recurring

Natural home remedy using baking soda:

1. Take some baking soda
2. Add water
3. Mix well to make a paste
4. Apply this paste on the infection

This will help dry up and heal the blisters.

Natural home remedy using black tea bags:

1. Take 1 cup of hot water
2. Put a black tea bag in it for 1-2 min
3. Allow the tea bag to cool

4. Place it on the sores for 5 min
5. Do this 3 times a day

The sores will crust and disappear naturally in 4-5 days.

Tips:

• Rub ice on the infected area to slow down the growth of cold sores
• Include yogurt in the diet as it stimulates the immune system and prevents cold sores

Prickly Heat
Treat prickly heat rashes with natural home remedies using chickpea flour or papaya.
Prickly Heat:

• Prickly heat is a skin condition caused by collection of sweat
• It occurs around body parts which are prone to sweating, like the:
  o Back
  o Underarms
  o Waist
  o Chest

Symptoms to look for:

- Rashes and raised bumps on the skin
- Intense itching

Causes:

- Sweat causes irritation of the skin

Natural home remedy using chickpea four and margosa leaves:

1. Take ½ bowl of chickpea flour
2. Add 15-20 crushed margosa leaves
3. Add little water to make a paste
4. Mix well
5. Apply on the affected area
6. Leave it for 15 min
7. Wash off with cold water

This removes the dead skin cells and provides relief from inflammation

Natural home remedy using papaya or cucumber:

1. Take some papaya or cucumber pulp
2. Apply on the affected area
3. Leave it for 25 min
4. Wash off with water

This cools the affected area and relieves the itching

Tips:

• To prevent rashes during summer:
  o Wear loose cotton clothes
  o They dry off easily

Hives
Treat hives with natural home remedies by using either pomegranate or margosa (neem) leaves.
Hives:

• Hives is also known as urticaria
• It refers to development of rashes on the skin

Symptoms to look for:

• Skin rashes, which are raised in shape
• Itching
• Burning sensation
• Rashes keep changing location on skin. They disappear from one area and appear on the other part
  after a while

Causes:

• When the skin comes in contact with an allergen or irritant, the body releases chemical called histamine.

The action of histamine on the blood vessels leads to reddish bumps

Natural home remedy using margosa leaves and giloy powder:

1. Crush 20-25 margosa leaves to make paste
2. Add this paste to about 300 ml of water
3. Add 1 tsp of giloy powder
4. Giloy powder is available at ayurvedic shops
5. Boil the water till its level reduces to half
6. Strain the liquid
7. Cool till lukewarm
8. Drink 3 times a day

Natural home remedy using pomegranate and Indian gooseberry:

1. Take ½ glass pomegranate juice
2. Add ½ glass Indian gooseberry juice
3. Mix the juices together
4. Drink 2 times day

Natural home remedy using corn starch and baking soda:

1. Take ½ tub of warm water

2. Add ½ cup corn starch
3. Add ½ cup baking soda
4. Mix well
5. Soak a towel in this water
6. Wipe yourself with this soaked towel at least once everyday

Scabies
Treat scabies with natural home remedies using either margosa leaves or drumsticks.
Scabies:

• Scabies is a skin condition
• It's a body's response to presence of certain species of mites

Symptoms to look for:

• Intense itching especially at night
• Skin rashes
• Blisters
• Red, dry, sore and swollen skin
Causes:

• Scabies is a contagious condition
• It can spread through:
  o Physical contact
  o Contact with bed linen or clothing of the patient

Natural home remedy using margosa leaves and mustard oil:

1. Crush 20-25 margosa leaves to paste
2. Add 2 tbsp mustard oil
3. Apply on the infected area
4. Leave it on for 1 hr
5. Wash off with cold water
6. Repeat every day till lesions are completely healed

Margosa kills mites and speeds up healing

Natural home remedy using drumsticks and sesame oil:

1. Chop and crush a couple of drumsticks
2. Press on a sieve and extract their juice
3. Add 2 tbsp sesame oil
4. Mix well
5. Apply on the infected area
6. Leave it for 20 min
7. Wash off with water

Drumsticks soothe irritation and itchiness

Chilblain

Treat chilblain with natural home remedies by using either onion or lemon.
Chilblains:

• Chilblains are painful, reddish swellings on the skin
• They occur due to exposure to excessive cold

Symptoms to look for:

• They usually occur on areas prone to becoming cold like:
  o Toes
  o Fingers
  o Nose
  o Ear lobes
• Sometimes it may affect:
  o Heels
  o Lower legs
  o Thighs

Causes:

• Blood vessels beneath the skin narrow when skin becomes cold
• Vessels expand when skin warms
• This leads to leakage from blood vessels causing chilblains

Natural home remedy using onion:

1. Take 1 bowl of crushed onion
2. Press it on a sieve and extract its juice
3. Apply juice on the affected area

Natural home remedy using potato and salt:

1. Take a potato slice
2. Sprinkle it with salt
3. Rub the salted side on the affected area

Natural home remedy using lemon:

1. Take juice of ½ lemon
2. Rub on affected toes and fingers

Tips:

• Massage your toes and fingers to improve blood circulation
• Wear warm clothes in cold weather
• Keep your head and ears warm
• Do not heat the skin immediately if you've been out in the cold

Shingles
Treat shingles with natural home remedies using either aloe vera leaves or liquorice.

Shingles:

• Shingles is caused by the chickenpox virus
• This virus usually affects a single nerve or 2-3 adjacent nerves on one side of the body

Symptoms to look for:

• Rashes on the skin
• Itchy blisters

Causes:

• The chicken pox virus stays dormant in the body
• The virus may multiply and affect the nerves years later
• The condition generally affects people with a poor immune system

Natural home remedy using aloe vera and honey:

1. Remove the thorns and outer skin from a few aloe vera leaves
2. Extract all the gel from inside
3. Take 1 bowl of this aloe vera gel
4. Add 1 tsp of honey
5. Mix well

6. Apply on the affected area 2 times a day

Natural home remedy using liquorice powder:

1. Take 1 tsp of liquorice powder
2. Add a little water
3. Mix well to make a paste
4. Apply on the affected area

Natural home remedy using garlic:

1. Crush 5-6 garlic cloves to paste
2. Apply this paste on the affected area
3. Leave it for 15 min
4. Wash off with water

Abrasion

Treat skin abrasions with natural home remedies using aloe vera leaves or turmeric. Abrasion:

• Abrasion refers to the damage to the upper layer of the skin
• It occurs when a friction force is applied on the skin

Symptoms to look for:

• Abrasion can be painful and can cause bleeding

Causes:

• Rubbing of skin against a rough surface
• Occurs if body is thrown strongly against an object
• Children often get scratches while playing

Natural home remedy using aloe vera:

1. Remove the thorns and outer skin of aloe vera leaves
2. Extract gel from inside
3. Apply this gel on the abrasion
4. Let it stay on the skin
5. Repeat this 3 times a day

Natural home remedy using turmeric:

1. Turmeric is an effective antiseptic
2. Take ½ tsp turmeric powder
3. Add a little water
4. Mix well to make a paste
5. Clean the abrasion with cotton
6. Apply turmeric paste on it
7. Allow it to dry on the skin
8. Do not cover the wound

9. Repeat this 3 times a day

• Clove powder may also be used instead of turmeric

Natural home remedy using milk and turmeric:

1. Take 1 cup of warm milk
2. Add ½ tsp of turmeric in it
3. Drink this every day
4. It strengthens the immune system and speeds up the healing process

Razor Burn
Treat razor burns with natural home remedies using either strawberries or aloe vera leaves.
Razor Burn:

• Shaving incorrectly or using a blunt razor can lead to razor burns

Symptoms to look for:

• Red rashes on the skin after shaving

Causes:

• Applying excessive pressure during shaving
• Lack of skin lubrication

• Shaving in the direction opposite of the hair growth

Natural home remedy using strawberries and fresh cream:

1. Crush 4-5 strawberries
2. Add 1 tbsp fresh cream
3. Mix well
4. Apply on the affected area
5. Leave for 10 min
6. Repeat 2 times a week to reduce irritation

Natural home remedy using aloe vera:

1. Remove thorns and outer covering of a few aloe vera leaves
2. Extract gel from inside
3. Apply the gel on the affected area

Tips:

• Use warm water for shaving as this softens the hair and makes it easier to shave
• Apply a moisturising cream on face 15 min before shaving

Bed Sores

Treat bed sores with natural home remedies by using either honey or aloe vera leaves.

Bed Sores:

• Bed sores is a common condition suffered by bed ridden people
• It affects the body parts which are under constant pressure due to a still body posture

Symptoms to look for:

• Blue, purple or dark patches on the affected body parts
• Ulcers and open wounds develop over time

Natural home remedy using beetroots and honey:

1. Wash and peel 3 beetroots
2. Slice and grind them to make a paste
3. Put the paste on a sieve and extract the juice
4. Add 2 tbsp of honey to this juice
5. Mix well
6. Apply on sores with cotton
7. Tie a clean bandage to avoid stains
8. Apply the mixture 2-3 times a day

Natural home remedy using honey and sugar:

1. Take 2 tbsp of honey
2. Mix 2 tbsp of sugar in it
3. Place this in a bowl of hot water
4. Apply on sores when solution becomes lukewarm

Natural home remedy using aloe vera:

1. Peel the outer green covering of an aloe vera leaf
2. Extract the gel from inside
3. Apply this gel on the sores
4. Rub gently for 2-3 minutes
5. Wipe with a clean damp cloth
6. Repeat 2-3 times a day

Tips:

• Change position of the patient regularly
• Use soft mattresses for the patient

Chafing
Treat chafing with natural home remedies by using either aloe vera or margosa (neem) leaves.
Chafing:

• Chafing refers to the skin irritation which occurs as a result of friction experienced by the skin

Symptoms to look for:

• Chafing usually occurs around the:
  o Inner thighs
  o Armpits
  o Nipples
  o Groin area
• The skin becomes tender and sore
• If neglected, chafing leads to bruising and infection

Causes:

• Rubbing of body parts with each other
• Poorly fitted underwear
• Usually athletes and obese people are prone to chafing

Natural home remedy using turmeric powder:

1. Take 3 tsp turmeric powder
2. Add 1 tsp water
3. Mix well to make paste
4. Apply paste on the affected area
5. Leave it for 30 min

6. Cover it with a cloth
7. Wash off with water

Natural home remedy using margosa leaves and lemon:

1. Crush a handful of margosa leaves
2. Squeeze ½ a lemon
3. Mix well to from a paste
4. Apply this paste on the affected area

Natural home remedy using aloe vera:

1. De-thorn and remove the outer skin of a few aloe vera leaves
2. Extract aloe vera gel from inside
3. Apply aloe vera gel on the affected area
4. Wash it off with water after 30 min
5. Wipe the area dry
6. Do this twice every day

Tips:

• Do not wear ill fitting underwear
• Keep the body lubricated by applying mustard oil on underarms and inner thighs
• Use baby powder on chafing prone areas

Measles

Treat measles with natural home remedies by using either basil leaves or fenugreek seeds
Measles:

• Measles is a highly contagious viral infection
• It commonly affects children
• Vaccination has reduced its occurrence in recent years

Symptoms to look for:

• Fever
• Sore eyes
• Runny nose
• Cough
• Sore throat
• Loss of appetite
• Skin rashes in form of round spots
   o They appear around face and neck and then spread to other parts of the body
   o Initially pink, the spots darken as the condition progresses

Causes:

• Incorrect eating habits
• Living in unhygienic conditions

Natural home remedy using:

1. Take 2 tsp crushed basil leaves
2. Press on a sieve and extract its juice
3. Add 1 tsp turmeric powder
4. Mix well
5. Consume 2 times a day

Natural home remedy using:

1. Soak 2 tbsp fenugreek seeds in 1 glass water
2. Leave it for 2 hr
3. Drink 3 tsp of this water every 30 min

Tips:

• Keep the patient in a separate and clean room till cured
• Do not share common objects like bed linen, towels etc. with the patient as this will prevent the
  infection from spreading

Bruises
Treat bruises with natural home remedies by using either garlic or spinach.
• When you fall or bump into something, some blood vessels get ruptured beneath the skin leading to
  collection of blood

• Bruises naturally heal within 2-3 weeks

Symptoms to look for:

• Black or blue discoloration of skin
• Sharp pain

Causes:

• Falls or bumps
• Bleeding disorders
• Leukaemia
• Scurvy

Natural home remedy using ice:

1. Wrap some ice in a piece of cloth
2. Apply this on the affected area
3. This reduces inflammation and pain
4. Apply heating pads after 2-3 hours
5. This will improve the blood circulation

Natural home remedy using garlic, onion, turmeric powder and mustard oil:

1. Crush 3-4 garlic cloves to a paste
2. Take 3 tsp of this paste
3. Add 3 tsp of chopped onion
4. Add 3 tsp turmeric powder

5. Add 2-3 tbsp of mustard oil
6. Mix well
7. Apply on the affected area

Natural home remedy using spinach:

1. Crush a handful of spinach leaves to a paste
2. Apply this paste on the affected area
3. Leave it for 20 min
4. Wash it off with normal water

Tips:

NEVER APPLY ICE DIRECTLY ON THE SKIN AS IT
CAN DAMAGE THE SKIN TISSUE

Chapter 9: Pre-Cleanse (Nighttime Only)

While Western skincare routines typically start out with you scrubbing your makeup off with a cleanser, the Korean alternative takes a much different approach. Pre-cleansing is basically unheard of in the West, but it is a very important step!

In the pre-cleansing step, you remove all of your makeup gently by using cleansing oil. "Gently" is definitely the keyword here! Korean women would be appalled to see how some Western women harshly scrub their faces with wash cloths in order to remove stubborn mascara.

Cleansing oils come in a variety of types; however, there are very few cleansing oils available on the Western market. Most likely, you will need to shop online for a Korean brand. You can choose one for dry skin, oily skin, brightening, or moisturizing, among many others. Assess your skin and choose a product that is tailored to your type.

You can opt for makeup wipes before using the cleansing oil, but it's really not necessary. If used properly, cleansing oil will take away most of your hard to remove makeup, including eye makeup.

In order to use cleansing oil properly, first ensure that your hands and face are completely dry. Take a pump or two of the oil and rub a light layer over your entire face. Massage the oil into your skin, using circular motions, for several minutes. Your face makeup should start to break up, making it really easy to wash off.

Next, massage some of the oil over your eyes to break up the eye makeup. Take your time here, and be extremely gentle. The skin around your eyes is very fragile. If you rub too harshly, you'll get premature wrinkles (or make any current wrinkles worse)!

Once you've finished with your eyes, it's time to emulsify the oil. Wet your hands with a bit of warm water, and pat it all over your face. You should use just a little bit of water at a time until you get the right amount. The oil should start to turn white or cloudy. Massage your skin again, ensuring the oil becomes emulsified all over. Finally, rinse your face off. Nearly all of your makeup should have come off with the cleansing oil. If there's still some residue left behind, don't worry—this is completely normal. The oil's main job is to gently remove the makeup so that you don't have to scrub it off.

Pre-cleansing is meant to be a part of your nighttime routine. Don't worry about this step in the morning!

167

Cleanse

Now you're ready to use a regular cleanser on your face. For your morning routine, this should always be your first step.

What type of cleanser you use is totally up to you; however, foaming cleansers are a popular choice for many Korean women. You may also find that gentle cream cleansers work well. Similar to oil cleansers, you can find many cream and foaming cleansers that are geared towards specific skin types and needs. Foam cleansers are usually the most gentle, so if you have sensitive skin, opt for a foam cleanser.

Many Western women use wash cloths or other abrasive materials to wash their faces. On the other hand, Korean women usually just use their fingers, as they are the mildest tools you can use. Again, the key here is to be very gentle; do not rub the product into your skin harshly. Instead, spread the foam or cream very lightly over your face. Then add some water, and rub softly in circular motions to buff away the rest of the makeup residue.

Rinse your face with warm water and pat to dry. Do not use a towel to dry your face!

If you notice any leftover eye makeup (such as eyeliner or mascara), simply dip a cotton swab into some makeup remover and gently swipe at the leftover makeup. This is also a good strategy to use if you are wary of getting oil cleansers or regular cleansers too close to your eyes. Most oil cleansers are safe to use on your eyes, but if it's easier for you, just use a cotton swab.

Exfoliate (nighttime only)

Exfoliators contain grains or microbeads that work to remove dead skin cells and other impurities from the skin. Good exfoliation is key for clear, soft, youthful-looking skin. Ensuring your skin is free of dead skin cells will help you look your best! If you do not exfoliate, the buildup of dead cells will make your skin look dull, tired, and dry. Your makeup will also look very patchy and cakey.

While exfoliation is definitely part of the Korean skincare routine, it is important to note that it is not a daily step. You should never exfoliate every day because over-exfoliation can dry your skin out and cause breakouts!

With a wide range of exfoliators available, it can be hard to know which one to choose. Sugar scrubs are typically gentle on the skin, but even people with sensitive skin can tolerate scrubs with microbeads if they are used gently. Many scrubs also contain natural ingredients such as rice and fruit extracts, making them extra healthy for your skin.

Typically, you should use an exfoliator one to two times a week. Any more than that, you're likely to damage your skin. If you think you need to exfoliate more than twice a week, try using the product just on areas that really need it (such as places where you have large pores or noticeable blackheads).

All exfoliators work the same; simply spread a generous amount of the product evenly onto your face and rub in circular motions. The grains will break up the dead skin cells, making them easy to rinse off. Massage around your face for around three to five minutes, paying special attention to places where you have the most problems (large pores, blackheads, acne, et cetera). Finally, rinse it all away with warm water to reveal fresh, super soft skin!

One area you should not overlook while exfoliating is your lips. Chapped lips can benefit greatly from some good exfoliation. You can purchase products that are specifically designed to be lip scrubs—this is safer than using a regular exfoliator on your lips, just in case you get some in your mouth! Use your finger to buff a lip exfoliator over your lips for a few minutes and watch the chapped skin fall away. Your lips will be much smoother and healthier looking.

Toner

Similar to the Western-style routine, the Korean routine also incorporates a toner. Toners from Korean brands contain different ingredients than your typical Western toners. Most Western brand toners are full of alcohol and other drying ingredients. Korean toners, on the other hand, do not contain alcohol and are meant to hydrate the skin.

There are actually several purposes of the toner step in the Korean skincare routine. The first is, as mentioned above, to hydrate the skin. Another purpose is to remove fine traces of residue from the first two steps. It's pretty clear—Korean women like to make absolutely sure their skin is squeaky clean (without being dried out, of course)!

Yet another purpose of the toner step is to soothe your skin. After using a Korean brand toner, your skin will feel very refreshed. This makes toner a wonderful step for your morning routine! The final purpose of the toner is to rebalance the pH level of your skin.

Toners come in many varieties, but it's unlikely you will find one that you react badly to, since Korean toners do not contain harsh chemicals. Most are marketed as "refreshers," so more likely than not, you'll end up with one that is great at hydrating and waking up the skin. You can also purchase a separate toner for use at nighttime. If you choose to do so, go for one that is meant to be soothing. However, you can certainly use the same toner in your morning and night routines.

Use a cotton pad or cotton ball to swipe the toner over your face. Let it air dry and absorb completely before moving on to the next step.

Essences

Applying an essence is one of the most essential steps to the Korean skincare routine. It is also one of the more unique steps, as Western skincare does not have this type of product.

Essences are liquid products that come either in the form of a lightweight lotion or a mist. Their purpose is to promote skin cell renewal, which helps keep your skin looking youthful and firm. If you have started to age, essences can help you regain some elasticity in your skin. Most essences will help you achieve a brighter, healthier looking complexion. (There are also many Korean products that claim to "whiten" the skin, but don't worry, essences will not bleach your skin).

You may want to try out several essences in order to find one that works best for you. Some Korean women use more than one!

If you use an essence in the form of a lotion, simply pat a thin layer on. If you opt for a mist instead, spray it all over your face and neck, patting it in afterwards. Let the essence completely absorb before you move on to the next step!

Ampoules

Ampoules may also be strange to you if you're unfamiliar with Asian beauty routines. Think of ampoules as similar to Western serums. They're a bit thicker and much more concentrated than essences. These products are usually the consistency of oil and often come in a jar with an eye dropper applicator.

Ampoules contain powerful vitamins, so a little bit of the serum goes a long way! They are meant to target your current skin issues such as dull complexion, loss of elasticity, wrinkles, and uneven skin tone.

Ampoules can also be used as a preventative measure. Even if you're young, you can still benefit from incorporating an ampoule into your skincare regimen. Use one to fight off the common signs of aging now, and you'll have less to worry about in the future. It's much easier to prevent than to correct!

You can mix and match your essences and ampoules, and it is very common for Korean women to use more than one of each! Do your research before purchasing essences and ampoules; look for ones that target the problems your skin currently has (or the problems you want to prevent). Everyone's skin is different, so we all have different needs. Create your own customized mix of essences and ampoules in order to treat your skin specifically. You can also rotate between different ampoules and essences in order to maximize your skin's benefits without having to slather on multiple ones every night.

Use the eye dropper tool (if your ampoule comes with one) to dispense a few drops of the product around your face. Then, spread the product evenly over your face and rub it in gently. Remember to let it absorb completely before moving on to the next step.

Moisturize

This step should look very familiar to you—moisturizing is an important part in almost any skincare routine, Korean or not. After cleansing your skin, especially as thoroughly as you will if you follow the Korean skincare routine, you're going to need to replenish your skin's moisture. Well-hydrated skin will stay healthy and youthful. As you age, your skin will need more and more moisture, so everyone's routine will look a little bit different here.

For your daytime routine, be sure to use a light moisturizing lotion. If you have oily skin, you can opt for a gel formula. If you have really dry skin, you should start out with a light moisturizer first. See if your skin reacts well to just a lightweight lotion; don't worry about adding in any additional moisture at first. However, if your skin isn't quite as hydrated as you'd like, replace your light lotion with a heavier one.

It's important to note that Korean brand lightweight moisturizers are not always called "lightweight moisturizers." Korean products sometimes get very creative with their names, so be aware that "milk," "emulsion," and "lotion," can all mean the same thing!

For your nighttime routine, you may choose to use anywhere from one to three moisturizers!

It's up to you, and you should base your routine off of your skin's needs.

The first type of moisturizer you can use at night is the same emulsion or lightweight lotion you use during the day. After that, you can put on a heavier night cream. Once that absorbs, topping it all off with a sleeping pack will ensure your skin will be completely moisturized all throughout the night! Sleeping packs are essentially thick moisturizers chockfull of beneficial (usually anti-aging) ingredients. Some sleeping packs require you to rub them in while others instruct you to layer it on with a brush. You then leave the pack on all night and wash it off in the morning for super hydrated, radiant skin. There are hundreds of sleeping packs on the market, all geared towards different needs.

Using three moisturizers at night may seem a bit excessive, but remember, Korean women are serious about their skincare! You can certainly get by with only using one moisturizer. If you choose to use only one, make it a heavy night cream, as they are better at keeping your skin hydrated while you sleep. You can also choose to add in a sleeping pack a few times a week instead of putting one on every night.

No matter how many moisturizers you put on, be sure to give them plenty of time to absorb before adding additional layers of moisture. If you're going to use a sleeping pack, make sure it's the last thing you put on!

Eye Creams

The eye cream step should be in both your daytime routine and your nighttime routine. The eye area is especially delicate and prone to wrinkles, so choose an eye cream that hydrates, prevents or treats signs of aging, and improves elasticity. You can get by with using one eye cream for both your morning and night routines, but keep in mind a lot of eye creams are thick. Thick eye creams don't fare the best under makeup, so you'll be better off using a thinner cream during the day. Save the thicker cream for nighttime when you need the most hydration!

Many Korean eye creams are multifunctional, so you can purchase one product that will brighten, prevent signs of aging, hydrate, improve elasticity, and treat puffiness all in one! You'll also notice a lot of interesting ingredients in Korean brand eye creams, such as snail extract. Extracts from bees (such as bee venom) are also common ingredients. Do not be alarmed! While it may sound gross to put snail slime and bee venom on your skin, these ingredients are actually very beneficial. Snail extract in particular is known to improve the elasticity of the skin, so if you want youthful looking under eyes, get over the gross factor!

It is often said that the Korean skincare industry is years ahead of the Western industry; it's true that they have really innovative and interesting products and ingredients that you just can't get on the Western market. While some things will certainly catch on, Korean brands will always have a uniqueness to them you can't come by elsewhere. Don't be alarmed if you see "weird" ingredients—just remember how advanced the Korean skincare industry is!

SPF (daytime only)

Most Koreans are crazy about sun protection. It is not uncommon to see women carrying umbrellas on sunny days, just to keep the sun off their skin. Others may wear visors or large hats. It's also common to see people covering their arms in order to avoid any exposure to the sun.

This may strike you as odd, since many Westerners desire tan skin, often lying around in the sun for hours in the summer or visiting tanning salons in order to fake the bronzed skin look. In Korea, it's totally the opposite. Pale skin is desirable, as traditionally it indicated that someone was from a rich family. Rich families stayed indoors while poor ones were forced to work outside in the sun, thus tanning their skin. Pale was always considered more beautiful than tan, and that mentality is still around in modern Korea.

For women in particular, sun protection is a huge concern. Most Korean BB creams and foundations contain a dose of SPF in order to cater to the market they serve. Even though these products already have SPF, many Koreans wear an additional regular sunscreen product on a daily basis!

There is a wide array of sunscreens in varying SPF levels available on the Korean market. You don't have to purchase a special Korean sunscreen if you don't want to; you can use a Western sunscreen brand, as there aren't any special ingredients in Korean sunscreens. What's most important is that the sunscreen is at least SPF 20 and blocks both UV-A and UV-B rays.

You should apply sunscreen every day, even if it's not sunny outside. The sun's rays can still penetrate through the cloud cover enough to cause a slight tan over a long period of time. What should be more of a concern, however, is that exposure to the sun (including on cloudy days) can cause premature signs of aging as well as skin cancer. You should be using a sunscreen as part of your daily skincare routine if you want to prevent both damage to your health and to your skin.

Although BB creams and foundations have SPF in them already, studies have shown that in order to benefit from the SPF in these products, you would have to use at least four times the amount of the product that you normally use. Since the SPF is not concentrated enough in the BB creams or foundations, you need to add an additional product (with the main function of this product being SPF) to your routine. Think of the SPF in BB creams and foundations as an extra shot of protection.

The best time to apply sunscreen is after you finish all of the other steps in your morning skincare routine, but before you apply any makeup (including face primers).

In addition to wearing sunscreen, large hats/visors or umbrellas, and long sleeves to protect their skin, Koreans also wear sunglasses often in order to protect the delicate skin around their eyes. Even though sunglasses aren't a skincare product, you should consider wearing them daily as part of your routine as well!

Masks & Facial Massages

This final chapter will detail a couple of steps that are considered to be "extra." These are steps in the Korean skincare routine that you don't have to perform every night, but they are still part of the routine and can be very beneficial to your skin. Some women do perform them almost every night, but they aren't as necessary as the other steps in the routine.

Masks

Face masks are something you will definitely see all over Korea. Not only are there several types of face masks to choose from (such as sheets masks, liquid masks, packs, and so on), there are also endless variations in scents, ingredients, and beneficial properties. There are masks that brighten, whiten, hydrate, cool, renew, and just about anything else under the sun!

You can purchase any type of mask you need in the form of a tube, jar, or sheet. Tubes usually contain masks that are more on the liquid side. Jars are for the thicker masks (such as clay masks), and sheet masks are thin slips of paper soaked in different essences.

Masks that come in tubes and jars are pretty self-explanatory—you simply apply the product to your face, allow it to dry, and wash it off with warm water. These are very similar to masks on the Western market, but of course many of them are geared towards different skin issues. For example, brightening and whitening masks are really common in Korea. It's important to note that "whitening" does not indicate bleaching! If you use a whitening mask over a long period of time, your skin may become a bit lighter, but it won't be anything drastic. Sometimes, "whitening" is used interchangeably with "brightening," even though these terms don't mean the same thing in English.

Sheet masks are sort of a novelty for those of us in the West. There are a few Western brands that have come out with sheet masks, but you certainly can't get the same kind of variety you can with the Korean sheet masks.

Sheet masks are a really convenient way to boost your skincare routine. These masks are packaged in individual sachets. All you have to do is remove the mask and place it over your face, lining up the eye and mouth holes in the paper. Press the mask until it adheres to your skin, and leave it on for about 20 minutes. You can leave it on for as long as you like, especially since the masks are always so saturated with essence! It takes them a long time to dry out. You can also use the leftover liquid in the packet to brush on your skin after you take the mask off. Let it absorb into your skin and carry on with your routine!

No matter what type of mask you use, it's best to use it after your toner. This way you won't be cleansing away all of the good ingredients the mask is putting into your skin! It's best to use masks once or twice a week, but if your skin is really problematic, you can use one three times a week. You may want to alternate between types of masks as well; this way you can treat your skin to different ingredients each time. For example, one night you can use a clay mask to remove impurities. A few nights later, you can use a brightening sheet mask to enhance your complexion. Finally, a cooling or hydrating mask is always a good idea! They can make a huge difference if used once a week.

Facial Massages

Conclusion

Thank you again for purchasing this book!
I hope this book was able to help you understand the Korean take on skincare and inspire you to take better care of your skin. You should be able to effectively adopt a Korean skincare routine now!
Thank you, and good luck!

www.ingramcontent.com/pod-product-compliance
Lightning Source LLC
Chambersburg PA
CBHW060331030426
42336CB00011B/1296